The Active Woman's Pregnancy Log

The Active Woman's Pregnancy Log

A DAY-BY-DAY DIARY AND GUIDE TO A FIT AND HEALTHY PREGNANCY

Suzanne Schlosberg & Liz Neporent, M.A.

HOUGHTON MIFFLIN COMPANY

Boston New York 2008

For information about permission to reproduce selections
from this book, write to Permissions, Houghton Mifflin Company,
215 Park Avenue South, New York, New York 10003.

www.houghtonmifflinbooks.com

Library of Congress Cataloging-in-Publication Data

Schlosberg, Suzanne.
The active woman's pregnancy log : a day-by-day diary and guide
to a fit and healthy pregnancy / Suzanne Schlosberg and Liz Neporent.
p. cm.
Includes bibliographical references.
ISBN 978-0-618-78594-0
1. Physical fitness for pregnant women. 2. Logbooks.
3. Pregnant women—Diaries. I. Neporent, Liz. II. Title.
RG558.7.S35 2008
618.2'44—dc22   2008006543

Printed in China

Illustrations by Laura Hartman Maestro
Book design by Lisa Diercks

C&C 10 9 8 7 6 5 4 3 2 1

Acknowledgments

From Liz:

To Jay, with much love and gratitude, and to my beautiful Skylar, thanks for all the great in utero material for this book!

From Suzanne:

As always, I owe my husband, Paul Spencer, a big kiss for his design work and his encouragement. And two big kisses to my boys, Toby and Ian. Welcome to the world, little lads!

Contents

Important Contacts

HUSBAND/PARTNER: _____

HOME: _____

OFFICE: _____

CELL: _____

E-MAIL: _____

OB-GYN/PRACTITIONER: _____

NAME OF PRACTICE: _____

WEBSITE: _____

PHONE: _____

E-MAIL: _____

ADDRESS: _____

ASSOCIATE/NURSE: _____

REPRODUCTIVE ENDOCRINOLOGIST/SPECIALIST: _____

NAME OF PRACTICE: _____

WEBSITE: _____

PHONE: _____

E-MAIL: _____

ADDRESS: _____

ASSOCIATE/NURSE: _____

Important Contacts

MIDWIFE: _____

NAME OF PRACTICE: _____

WEBSITE: _____

PHONE: _____

E-MAIL: _____

ADDRESS: _____

BIRTHING SUPPORT: _____

CONTACT I: _____

NAME OF PRACTICE: _____

WEBSITE: _____

PHONE: _____

E-MAIL: _____

ADDRESS: _____

CONTACT 2: _____

NAME OF PRACTICE: _____

WEBSITE: _____

PHONE: _____

E-MAIL: _____

ADDRESS: _____

Important Contacts

PHARMACY:

CONTACTS:

WEBSITE:

PHONE:

E-MAIL:

ADDRESS:

LAB:

CONTACTS:

WEBSITE:

PHONE:

E-MAIL:

ADDRESS:

HOSPITAL:

CONTACTS:

WEBSITE:

PHONE:

E-MAIL:

ADDRESS:

x

Important Contacts

INSURANCE COMPANY: _____

ID # AND GROUP: _____

CONTACTS: _____

WEBSITE: _____

PHONE: _____

E-MAIL: _____

ADDRESS: _____

MASSAGE THERAPIST: _____

PHONE: _____

E-MAIL: _____

ADDRESS: _____

OTHER: _____

PHONE: _____

E-MAIL: _____

ADDRESS: _____

OTHER: _____

PHONE: _____

E-MAIL: _____

ADDRESS: _____

Introduction

Congratulations!

Actually, make that double congratulations: not only are you pregnant, but you're lucky enough to be with child in the era of the prenatal Pilates class and the maternity workout unitard.

Back when our moms were pregnant with us, "prenatal exercise" meant putting on men's pants and propping your feet up for nine months. Obstetricians, fearful that exercise might somehow harm the growing baby, discouraged pregnant women from breaking a sweat. In fact, in the 1950s, the medical establishment recommended that pregnant women walk no more than one mile a day, broken up into several sessions! Even as late as 1985, the American College of Obstetricians and Gynecologists recommended that women limit their workouts to 15 minutes and never allow their heart rates to creep above 140 beats per minute.

But all that has changed, and in a big way. Doctors now encourage their pregnant patients to work out at least three times a week, preferably more. That's because research has proven that prenatal exercise is not only safe for most pregnant women but also — when doctor approved — actually advantageous. As numerous studies show, prenatal exercise does not increase the risk for miscarriage, and it offers a wide range of health benefits for mom and even for baby. For example, women who exercise regularly throughout pregnancy

➡ have a lower risk of gestational diabetes and high blood pressure

➡ experience fewer aches and pains and take fewer back pain–related sick days from work

➡ gain on average 7 pounds less than pregnant women who don't exercise, yet still are well within normal ranges for weight gain

➡ have a more positive body image than women who don't work out

➡ may experience a lower rate of preterm delivery

➡ tend to have easier and shorter labors than sedentary women, lowering the risk of complications for mom and baby

➡ tend to deliver babies who have less body fat at birth, which may translate to a lower risk of diabetes and high blood pressure later in life

➡ recuperate more quickly after delivery

➡ typically weigh the same five years after pregnancy as they did before, whereas nonexercisers tend to weigh at least 10 pounds more

You may already be aware of many of these benefits, but from our experiences — Liz's rollercoaster pregnancy with her daughter, Skylar, and Suzanne's 36 weeks carrying her twin boys, Toby and Ian — knowing isn't as easy as doing. This is especially true when you're so nauseated that the mere mention of a Hamburger Helper TV commercial makes you queasy (that was Liz), or you're so wiped out that it's an effort to press the buttons on the remote (that was Suzanne in her first trimester).

You might also have concerns about how much and what type of exercise is advisable — is it really OK to do abdominal exercises during that crucial first trimester? — or wonder how to modify your workouts to keep you and your baby absolutely safe. Plus, as both of us learned, you may need to adjust your entire workout mindset; pregnancy is a time to let go of your usual goals and shift to more relaxed expectations, accepting and embracing the transformation of your body.

From start to finish, pregnancy poses challenges to staying active, but you can absolutely overcome these challenges! That's where this log comes in handy. Consider it your healthy pregnancy headquarters, a portable, one-stop source of inspiration, information, and organizational tools to keep you feeling fit and confident and exercising wisely throughout this amazing journey.

FOUR BOOKS IN ONE

The Active Woman's Pregnancy Log is all about maintaining an active pregnancy, but it's actually four books in one.

A FIT PREGNANCY GUIDE

The first section explains the benefits of prenatal exercise and offers trimester-by-trimester advice on strength training, cardiovascular exercise, and relaxation. You'll find the official exercise guidelines from the American College of Obstetricians and Gynecologists, along with our own, more extensive workout recommendations based on the latest research, expert advice, and our own experience. We also offer tips for working around the most problematic pregnancy symptoms, from morning sickness to heartburn to swollen feet, as well as a comprehensive workout routine adjusted for each trimester. Plus we give essential nutrition guidelines to keep your baby well nourished and to keep you feeling satisfied and at a healthy weight.

Of course, since every pregnancy is unique, it's essential to consult with your doctor about the workout and nutrition guidelines best suited for you. If you are carrying twins or higher-order multiples or are in another high-risk category, the guidelines here may need to be modified substantially.

A DAILY DIARY

The book's key feature is a daily journal, lasting a full 40 weeks, that will motivate you to stay active and eat healthfully, remind you to back off from exercise when your body says so, and encourage you to relax and reflect on your pregnancy and your life. With the vat of hormones being dumped into your system on a daily basis, noting the physical and emotional changes you're experiencing will help you work through the bad days and appreciate the wonderful ones. Jotting down your physical and emotional low points can be cathartic, and having a record of your high points will help you relive the memories of what life was like before waddling became your main mode of travel.

Liz's pregnancy journal reflects all sorts of ups and downs, especially during the third trimester, when she was feeling like she needed a "wide load" sign just to cross the street. Toward the end of her seventh month, Liz went jogging with her cousin Margie. Margie was so winded from keeping pace with her that she finally had to beg Liz to dial it down. Noted in Liz's log that day: "Have achieved the finest moment of my pregnancy!"

Alas, the glory was short-lived. A month later, Liz struggled through a 20-minute run, then stepped up onto a curb and felt like her kneecap had exploded. Her log notation that day: "Time to hang up the Nikes until after the baby."

For Suzanne, maintaining a log helped her figure out what — and when — to eat so she wouldn't keep waking up ravenous in the middle of the night. Early in her pregnancy, she filled her diary with notes like "Ate giant burrito at 8:30 P.M. and still woke up STARVING at 3 A.M.!!!" By experimenting with different foods and tracking her eating and sleeping habits, she finally solved the mystery: it was cottage cheese mixed with salsa and avocado, eaten at 10 P.M., that enabled her to get a good night's sleep. Not only was Suzanne relieved, but so was her sleep-deprived husband.

AN ORGANIZER/RECORD KEEPER

Even if you were voted "most likely to multitask" by your high school graduating class, you might still feel overwhelmed — with all the baby supplies to buy, the classes to take, the appointments to keep. To help you prepare as thoroughly as you can, we've provided numerous charts and checklists, including a list of key prenatal workout gear, a form for recording test results and doctor's visits, and a rundown of how to pack for the big day. When both your bladder and your breasts are leaking (this happened to Liz at her baby shower), it's also important to feel like you're in control of *something* in your life. Taking notes, staying organized, ticking off boxes as you work through a list — these are actions that can leave you feeling as empowered as Erin Brockovich even as your little uterine invader hijacks a good portion of your bodily functions.

A REMINDER AND A KEEPSAKE

Keep this log on your nightstand, toss it in your purse when you head to the doctor or your birthing class, and whip it out for reference when you're shopping for maternity cycling shorts online. After the big day comes and you arrive home with your bundle — or bundles! — of joy, tuck your log away for safekeeping. You never know: if you get pregnant again, the notes you made during this pregnancy might inspire you to keep active the next time around, when life is even busier and more complicated. If you're sure this is your final pregnancy, you'll still have a wonderful keepsake — a reminder of how dedicated you were to your own health, and your baby's, even when you could no longer see your feet on the treadmill.

Active Pregnancy Guide

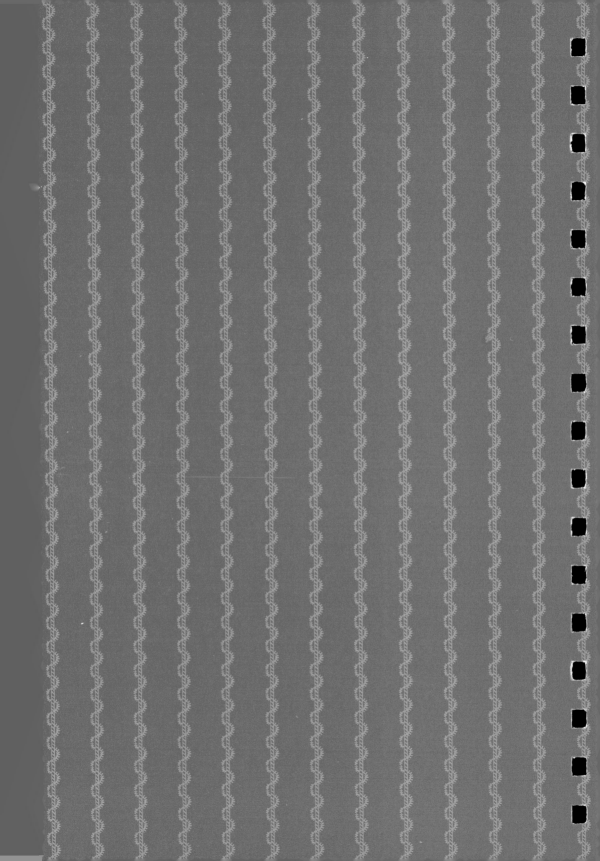

A Quick Guide to an Active Pregnancy

Sure, you could use pregnancy as an excuse to kick up your feet, eat cupcakes, and get reacquainted with *All My Children*'s Erica Kane. But that's not you. Whether you're the queen of your kickboxing class or a sofa spud ready to get off her duff so it doesn't expand to the size of her belly, you know that exercising while you're pregnant has countless benefits.

In this section, you'll find a rundown of these benefits, along with sensible advice on how to stay strong, keep up your stamina, and reach for your toes throughout the entire nine months. Plus we give tips for dealing with common pregnancy symptoms so they don't knock you out of the game, as well as eating advice to help your baby keep growing on schedule.

WHY PRENATAL EXERCISE IS SO GOOD FOR YOU — AND YOUR BABY

Back in the day when your mom was pregnant with you, the medical world tended to send the message that pregnancy was a grave disease; women who "caught it" weren't supposed to let their hearts pump too hard or work up a sweat beyond a dewy glisten. You were almost left with the impression that you'd be harming your baby, or yourself, if you walked for more than 20 minutes a day.

But many decades of research have shown conclusively that those fears were unfounded. Not everyone has gotten the update; your great-aunt Beverly might scold you for lifting anything heavier than the yellow pages, and you even may field warnings from strangers at the gym about "boiling your baby" while on the elliptical machine. Ignore these people! As long as you have your health practitioner's blessing to exercise, you can rest assured that you're doing the right thing.

While no one recommends that pregnant women compete in snowboard racing or sprint up the 1,575 steps of the Empire State Building, research shows that even relatively high levels of exercise are safe for fit moms-to-be who are pregnant with singletons. (There are no published studies on prenatal exercise during twin pregnancy, so ask your doctor for advice.) Numerous studies have been conducted on athletes and avid exercisers who have worked out five days a week for 30 to 90 minutes at moderate to high intensities practically until they were wheeled into the delivery room. If exercise were to cause any harm to mom or baby, the risks would have surfaced by now. Yet even among serious joggers and aerobics enthusiasts, no problems have been detected — not an increased risk of miscarriage, birth defects, injury to mom, premature labor, or stunted baby growth. Other studies have been conducted on less fit women who start a more moderate workout program during pregnancy, and exercise has been shown to be safe for these women, too.

How can this be? Won't all that huffing and puffing on the treadmill deprive your baby of oxygen? Won't your exercising thigh muscles hog up the blood supply that's supposed to be nourishing your baby? Won't all that sweating cause your little one to overheat?

Actually, no. It turns out that the changes your body undergoes during pregnancy serve to protect both mom and baby from harm during exercise. For example, research shows that a pregnant woman has a souped-up ability to eliminate the extra heat that's generated during exercise; in fact, when pregnant, you can generate about 20 percent more heat without causing your body temperature to rise. As long as you stay well hydrated and avoid insanely long, hard workouts or hot, humid temperatures (so unless you're an elite athlete, forget about running the Honolulu marathon), you needn't worry about spiking your baby's temperature.

Don't fret, either, that your baby's blood supply will be siphoned away to your muscles when you work out. Pregnant exercisers have blood volumes 10 to 15 percent higher than do pregnant couch potatoes, so when you're cranking away on the stationary bike, there's still plenty of blood flowing to your baby via the placenta. Know, too, that prenatal exercise stimulates the growth and function of the placenta, protecting the baby from oxygen deprivation.

Of course, now is not the time to aim for a personal-best in the 10k or to take up sports that require stellar balance, such as rock climbing or surfing. But as long as you use common sense and eat enough to compensate for the extra calories you're burning through exercise, you needn't worry that your workouts will compromise your baby's health or development.

Now that researchers have confirmed the safety of prenatal exercise, they've turned their focus to the benefits. Perhaps the biggest bonus is simply how you feel. Exercising moms-to-be are much less prone to back pain, leg cramps, and other nagging discomforts, and possibly carpal tunnel syndrome, sciatica, hemorrhoids, and constipation. And just like exercisers who aren't with child, pregnant exercisers are less likely to catch the flu or a cold.

You get a big psychological boost from prenatal exercise, too. Women of all fitness levels who work out during pregnancy report feeling happier about their burgeoning bodies, rather than regarding them as mystifying blobs. They also report more confidence going into labor. The most fit, active pregnant women — those who do aerobic exercise for 45 minutes five days a week — also tend to have shorter labors, perhaps up to one-third shorter, than other women, as well as a reduced need for interventions such as forceps, epidurals, and epi-siotomies and possibly even C-sections. Of course, even world-class athletes experience labors more grueling than an Olympic heptathlon, so even if the odds favor quicker, easier deliveries for fit women, there are no guarantees when it comes to childbirth.

Whether or not you sail through labor and delivery, if you exercise through-out pregnancy, you're likely to arrive at the big day at a healthy weight — rather than carrying excess poundage — and you're much more likely than sedentary women to return, eventually, to your prepregnancy weight. In a study of women who exercised through two pregnancies, the moms were on average lighter and leaner before their second pregnancy than before their first — precisely the opposite pattern of sedentary women.

It's more likely that your little one will be a lean, mean fighting machine, too. You might think that babies of exercising pregnant women would be at risk for low birthweight, but studies show they tend to weigh about the same as other babies. The only difference is that they carry less body fat, which may pay off years down the road in the form of lower risk of cardiovascular disease. At this point, the babies of exercising moms haven't been followed long enough for us to know for sure. However, in studies that have tracked the off-spring of exercising moms for five years, the babies were still less fat, heading into kindergarten, than the babies of women who didn't work out.

The bottom line: if you're having a low-risk pregnancy, exercise won't harm you or your baby and is likely to do both of you a world of good. But not every-one gets the green light to work out during these nine months. If your exercise program gets derailed due to preterm labor or because you're pregnant with triplets, follow your doctor's orders, and cut yourself some slack. The same advice applies if you find that you simply feel too nauseous or uncomfortable to work out as often as you'd planned. In the scheme of things, pregnancy is just a blip of time; once your baby enters the world, you'll have plenty of opportunity to get yourself back in shape.

OFFICIAL PRENATAL EXERCISE GUIDELINES

When the American College of Obstetricians and Gynecologists (ACOG) revised its prenatal exercise guidelines in 1994, the medical establishment finally lightened up. In fact, like most other medical and health expert sources, ACOG now strongly recommends that women stay active throughout their pregnancies.

That said, every pregnancy is an individual experience. Check with your doctor before starting or continuing any exercise routine, and keep her abreast of your workouts as your pregnancy progresses. These guidelines are an excellent start, but you may need to adjust them if health complications arise.

AMERICAN COLLEGE OF OBSTETRICIANS AND GYNECOLOGISTS (ACOG) GUIDELINES FOR EXERCISING WHILE PREGNANT

(From ACOG Technical Bulletin, Number 189, February 1994, with an update from the ACOG Committee Opinion on Exercise During Pregnancy and the Postpartum Period, Number 267, January 2002)

1. In the absence of either medical or obstetric complications, 30 minutes or more of moderate exercise a day on most, if not all, days of the week is recommended for pregnant women.

2. Don't exercise in the supine position (flat on your back) after the first trimester. This can decrease the blood flow to the uterus. Also, don't stand motionless for long periods.

3. Stop exercising when fatigued, and don't exercise to exhaustion. You might be able to continue doing weight-bearing exercise at close to your usual intensity throughout pregnancy, but non-weight-bearing activities, such as cycling and swimming, are easier to continue and carry less risk of injury.

4. Don't do exercises in which you could lose your balance, especially in the third trimester. Avoid any exercise that risks even mild abdominal trauma.

5. You need an additional 300 calories a day during pregnancy, so if you're exercising, be particularly careful to ensure an adequate diet. (Note: Despite ACOG's guidelines, many experts advise limiting the extra intake to 150 calories for the first two trimesters and 300 calories for the final three months.)

6. During the first trimester, be sure that you stay cool when exercising. Drink enough water, wear breathable clothing, and don't work out in too hot an environment.

7. After you give birth, resume your prepregnancy exercise routine gradually, based on your physical capacity.

UNOFFICIAL — BUT ESSENTIAL — EXERCISE GUIDELINES

The ACOG guidelines provide a starting point, but there's plenty more to know about prenatal exercise. Below are nine additional guidelines based on published research, interviews with exercise physiologists and medical doctors, and our own experience. These rules apply from the minute the stick turns blue.

1. Drink plenty of fluids before, during, and after each workout.

2. Don't rely on your heart rate as an indicator of how hard you're working out. When you're pregnant, your resting and exercise heart rates are higher than normal due to increased body temperature and a flood of hormones. Even if you have plenty of experience with heart-rate hardware, you'll have off-kilter readings right from the get-go. A more useful way to gauge prenatal exercise intensity is to use the RPE (rate of perceived exertion) scale: simply rate your exertion on a scale of 1 to 10, 10 being an all-out effort you can't sustain. Aim for an RPE of 4 to 7. A 4 feels like you're working moderately hard but could keep up the pace for quite a while without getting tired; at a 7, you feel like you could keep going for 30 minutes but no longer. A simpler option is to use the "talk test": if you can't carry on a conversation, you need to slow your pace. Stop immediately if you feel dizzy, fatigued, or experience vaginal bleeding.

3. Avoid exercising outdoors on very hot and humid days. Work out in the early morning or in the evening when it's cooler, or opt for an indoor workout.

4. Wear supportive athletic shoes designed specifically for your chosen activity (for example, walking shoes for walking, cross-trainers for weight

training), and invest in a good sports bra. At some point, you'll probably need shoes that are one-half to one size larger and a bra that's at least one size larger than normal.

5. If you're exercising outdoors, sun protection is more important than ever. Raging hormones increase the chance of developing dark patches of skin. Wear sunscreen and a protective hat.

6. Always warm up before a workout and cool down afterward. Both are essential for regulating your body temperature. Do at least 5 minutes of easy activity like walking, gentle calisthenics, or swimming at the front and back ends of your workout.

7. Monitor your center of gravity; it grows more off-kilter with every pound you gain and every inch your belly pooches outward. Avoid walking down steep hills or any activity that puts you at risk for falling.

8. Eat a small snack before exercise to avoid crashing and burning due to low blood sugar, a common occurrence for some pregnant women.

9. Avoid overstretching. Your hormones are working overtime, softening and loosening up your ligaments, so don't go beyond the normal range of motion or jar your joints with high-impact moves.

EXERCISE TIPS BY TRIMESTER

A brisk walk doesn't feel much different when you're five weeks pregnant than before you conceived, but when you're eight months along, tying your shoes may feel like a brisk walk. It's not just that the baby is growing outward, blocking your view beyond the very tip of your toes; during that last month before the baby pops out, you'll find it harder to breathe, your achy back will make it more challenging to bend over, and you may even find your wrists or fingers too swollen to grasp the laces. The bottom line: to keep up with your expanding, stretching, changing body and to ensure the safety of your little gumdrop-to-be, you'll need to modify your workouts as you venture toward the big day.

We've broken up the exercise guidelines by trimester because that's pretty much the schedule on which you'll find yourself needing to make changes.

EXERCISING IN THE FIRST TRIMESTER

For many women, exercise during the first three months of pregnancy is business as usual. Others experience such debilitating symptoms that they find themselves inconsolable after hearing about the possibility of rain in the morning weather report, or they can barely muster the energy to get out of bed before 3 P.M., let alone hit the gym.

Even for women who experience morning sickness, depression, and those other charming symptoms common during the first trimester, there are very few exercises or activities you absolutely need to avoid during these months, although common sense dictates avoiding skydiving and tackle football. Still, if you find yourself feeling winded or lethargic, you may need to divide your exercise into 10-minute mini-workouts. Even 10 minutes of activity will usually make you feel better, and you won't get out of the exercise habit.

What about the risk of miscarriage? While it's true that miscarriage risk is highest in the first three months, there's simply no evidence that exercise increases this risk and plenty of research to suggest that exercise does not. The majority of miscarriages are caused by genetic abnormalities of the embryo or a preexisting disease or other condition related to the mother. These are unfortunate situations that 45 minutes on the treadmill won't change.

Nonetheless, there are a few tweaks you should make to your program even before your bump is obvious.

STRENGTH TRAINING

▶ **Lighten up your weights.** You may be perfectly capable of hoisting 50-pound sacks of grain over your head or out-bench-pressing the boys, but when those pregnancy hormones flood your system, your joints are looser and less stable and you may be at greater risk of injury. The bummer — and the real surprise for women who've lifted weights on a regular basis — is that something as simple as lifting a book off the floor can lead to strained abdominal ligaments. So whether you're using free weights, machines, or exercise bands, decrease the resistance and increase your repetitions to 12 to 20 reps per set.

There are some exercises that just may not work for you at all, so pay careful attention to how your muscles respond to weight training, particularly the part of the muscle closest to the joint. Sometimes you don't even feel pain. You feel this weird sort of slipping or loosening near the joint, and then it goes *ping*. When you feel that, you need to stop. Reevaluate each time you work out; as you move through the weeks, months, and trimesters, you may need to adjust your routine.

➡ **Consider switching to Pilates or yoga.** You needn't lift a weight to get your muscle-toning fix; Pilates and yoga can help you stay strong even though there's no iron involved. Both are safe to do while you're pregnant as long as the routine conforms to pregnancy guidelines. (For example, hot yoga classes are a big no-no. Your body is working hard enough to regulate your body temperature <u>without</u> exercising in 100-degree heat.) Consider a class or private training sessions geared toward pregnant women.

➡ **Focus on breathing properly.** Inhale through your nose when you exert an effort, such as when you curl a dumbbell or pull the seated-row bar toward you, and exhale through your mouth when you release. Avoid exhaling forcefully without actually blowing out air, a mistake in technique known as the "Valsalva maneuver." While it's never a good idea, doing a Valsalva when you're pregnant puts you at risk for fainting, blood pressure spikes, and pelvic injuries.

CARDIO

➡ **Beginners:** Even if you weren't exactly an aerobic animal before you got pregnant, there's no reason you can't begin a cardio program now, as long as your healthcare expert gives you the thumbs-up. A basic walking program is a good place to start. Walk for 30 minutes two or three times per week, with a day of rest in between.

➡ **Intermediates:** If you were exercising for at least 90 minutes to 3 hours a week for at least three months prior to your pregnancy, you can continue the same routine three or four times a week, with a day of rest in between.

➡ **Advanced and athletes:** If you feel like you can continue your typical routine, go for it. Just pay attention to your body and obey its commands to back off or slow down, especially if you're accustomed to doing high-intensity interval training. (All-out intervals are not a good idea.) Priority number one is keeping you and the baby healthy. This is not the time to prove how tough you are. Whatever your fitness level, remember that heart rate isn't always the best indicator of how hard your body is working. See the exercise guidelines on page 5 for better intensity gauges.

STRETCHING AND RELAXATION

For the most part, you can carry on as usual with a stretching or yoga routine at this point in your pregnancy. Even if you're a flexibility neophyte, it will probably feel good to do something stretchy and mellow. Just don't push past your normal range of motion or to the point of discomfort. You're more likely to overstretch than before you got pregnant since the hormones responsible for loosening up your joints for labor have already begun to kick in.

Now is also a good time to start practicing meditation and deep breathing. You really will use these practices during labor, so the more experience you have, the better. Meditation doesn't mean you'll have to don long, flowing robes or stop shaving your legs. Find 5 to 15 minutes a day to sit in a quiet, un-cluttered space. Dim the lights, breathe deeply, unwind, and try to clear your mind. You might also want to try the traditional practice of repeating a mantra. Some women find it helpful to listen to music or soak in a bubble bath while meditating or simply relaxing.

SECOND TRIMESTER

As the little life form inside of you continues its takeover bid for your body, you should begin to make significant modifications to your exercise program. You may still be able to exercise relatively comfortably, but this is the point to put some extra precautions into place. One happy fact: women who feel lousy during their first trimester almost always get a reprieve from whatever symptoms plagued them once they hit the second-trimester milestone. Often they get this second wind virtually overnight.

STRENGTH TRAINING

➡ **Avoid lifting weights while standing still in one position for too long.** Because your blood volume increases to support the baby, remaining stationary for more than a few minutes at a time can cause blood to pool in your legs, leaving you feeling lightheaded and dizzy. Consider sitting or kneeling when you lift, walk around between sets, or use a workout ball as your bench.

➡ **Avoid lying on your back for too long.** Don't lie on a flat bench or on the floor to strength train, and don't get into any position that leaves your abdomen vulnerable to a falling weight. The heft of your expanding uterus can compress major blood vessels and restrict circulation, making you feel lightheaded and compromising blood flow to your ever-growing baby. This makes an even stronger case for doing weights while seated, kneeling, or on a ball. Do your abdominal exercises in a standing position, with your back against the wall, or perched on a workout ball. For any exercise you feel you must do lying down, don't stay in that position for more than a few minutes, especially if you begin to feel lightheaded. Or, try the move while lying on your side.

➡ **Bust out that new bra.** Your milk glands have begun to pump milk into your breasts, so they'll get larger. Enjoy your newfound voluptuousness, but give it some extra support. Buy a good sports bra that has a high percentage of Lycra and is at least one size larger than normal. Lycra shorts and tops that support your bump can be a huge help.

CARDIO

➡ **Beginners:** If you began a fitness routine in the first trimester, it's OK now to slightly increase your workout intensity. Here's a sample workout: warm up with a brisk 5- to 10-minute walk, then pick up the pace and power walk for 25 minutes while pumping your arms. Cool down by walking slowly for 5 minutes.

➡ **Intermediates:** If everything went well in your first trimester and you are feeling up to it, you can continue at the same pace.

➡ **Advanced and athletes:** Continue your routine if you're still comfortable, but stick to flat terrain to avoid any unintended adventures in gravity as your burgeoning belly throws you off-kilter. Decrease your workout duration or intensity if you're starting to feel like it's too much. On the other hand, if you were flattened by morning sickness in your first trimester, you might now find yourself exercising longer and at a higher level without extra effort.

Cross-train to maintain your fitness level and to help ease any joint problems that are beginning to surface. Even if you're feeling tiptop, it's a good idea to vary your workouts; that way, if one machine or activity suddenly becomes uncomfortable later in your pregnancy, your body already will be accustomed to the alternatives.

STRETCHING AND RELAXATION

Although your joints are bendier at this point, stretch with caution. Once ligaments overstretch, they won't snap back, and if you're too aggressive, your joints will remain unstable long after the baby is born. For meditation, prop yourself up with several large, fluffy pillows if sitting or kneeling for long periods of time has become uncomfortable.

THIRD TRIMESTER

You may have run like a gazelle or broken boards with your bare hands before you got pregnant, but now you're at your fattest and slowest. That's OK! If you can still waddle, you can work out. In addition to following all of first- and second-trimester rules, add the new precautions below. From here on, take it one day at a time. You may find that you'll be able to exercise until the day you give birth, but then again, there may come a point where putting on your sports bra feels like high-intensity interval training. Don't sweat the days you can't sweat too much. Remember that you're sharing your body now, so your tiny little bundle of joy also gets a vote in how you move and feel. Take solace in the fact that you've got the rest of your life to regain your fitness once you pop this kid out.

STRENGTH TRAINING

➡ **Avoid twisting or inverted movements.** At this point, you won't be able to do anything that involves twisting from the waist or bending over all the way. This will probably mean making additional edits to your abdominal, yoga, and Pilates workouts.

➡ **Watch your joints.** You expected your knees and lower back to ache, but your wrists and elbows? Excess fluid may cause carpal tunnel syndrome and other completely unexpected—and annoying—joint problems. Don't do anything that makes your joints go ping. See "Working Around Your Pregnancy Symptoms" on page 22 for tips on mitigating joint discomfort.

➡ **Limit getting up and down.** Even kneeling or sitting may become a challenge since your big belly will make it completely awkward to hoist yourself up from those positions. At this point, you will probably want to do all of your muscle toning from a standing position, keeping in mind that you shouldn't stand still for too long. To relieve back or hip pain, try placing one foot up on a box or step bench. Many women do better if they switch to exercise bands instead of weights from this point on, since it's easier to transition from exercise to exercise.

CARDIO

➡ **Beginners:** Aim to power walk for at least 30 minutes, but if you aren't up to it because of joint pain or because you're easily winded, try a machine with less impact, such as the stationary bike, stairclimber, or elliptical. Or, walk on a treadmill so you can cheat by leaning on the handrails a bit. Your hips may not feel as stable as they did in the second trimester, and your center of gravity has definitely shifted, so stick to level terrain. Continue to do cardio at least twice a week for as long as you can.

➡ **Intermediates:** Continue your routine if you are still comfortable, but stick to flat terrain. Decrease your mileage or workout time if moving becomes difficult; cross-train to maintain your fitness level.

➡ **Advanced and athletes:** Yes, some women do run right up until the moment they check into the hospital, but the majority of us will need to slow down and lighten up. For some, even walking may be too stressful on the hips, knees, or feet near the end, and swimming or water aerobics may be the best choice. Even if water exercise isn't normally your thing, give it a try. You may find yourself the lone pregnant woman in a pool of senior citizens, but no matter; you can't trip and fall, you won't feel like a big clod, and the sense of weightlessness feels sooooooooooo good. At the very end of your pregnancy, you may need to take a week off and put your feet up, which is perfectly fine. Know that you've earned the rest and can always get back up to speed once your baby is on the outside.

STRETCHING AND RELAXATION

Stretching and yoga will help you stay calm and offer some joint-ache relief, but don't overdo it, and make the appropriate modifications. Even a motion as simple as reaching for your toes while sitting on a chair will probably be impossible toward the end. But you may still be able to do some stretches from a standing position while holding on to the back of a chair or the wall for support. If you've neglected to rehearse your breathing techniques, it's not too late to start. Any practice will help you through the labor process.

MUST-DO STRENGTH EXERCISES

You can continue strength training throughout your pregnancy. In fact, staying strong will help you support the extra weight of the baby when she's on the inside as well as when she's finally on the outside. Although you can continue to work every muscle in your body straight through the ninth month, you'll need to do some tweaking — and some outright overhauling — of certain moves. For example, it's obvious that you can't pull off a stomach crunch three days before you give birth, but there's still a way to continue work on your abs.

Refer to the chart on page 22 for suggestions on some excellent muscle-toning and strengthening exercises to do at each stage of your pregnancy. Of course, there are plenty of other strength moves you can do, but these are some of the most tried and true exercises for pregnant women. Check with an expert about any move you're unsure is safe during pregnancy.

CRUNCHLESS CRUNCH

Benefit: Strengthens the core muscles of your abs and lower back.

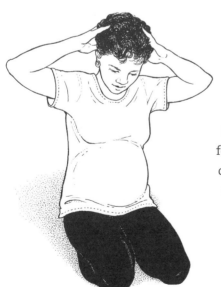

[A] Lie face-up with your knees bent and feet hip-width apart and flat on floor. Place your palms just below and on either side of your belly button, pressing down firmly.

[B] Tighten your abdominal muscles in and downward. When your muscles feel fully engaged, hold for 15 seconds, continuing to breathe normally. Do 1–2 sets, 5–10 reps per set.

KNEELING CRUNCHLESS CRUNCH

Do the Crunchless Crunch in a kneeling position.

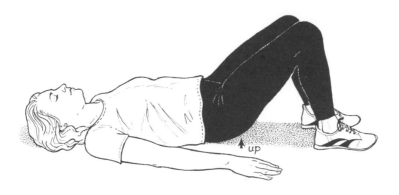

PELVIC TILT

Benefit: Strengthens your pelvic floor muscles.

[A] Lie face-up with your knees bent, feet hip-width apart and flat on floor, and arms relaxed at your sides.

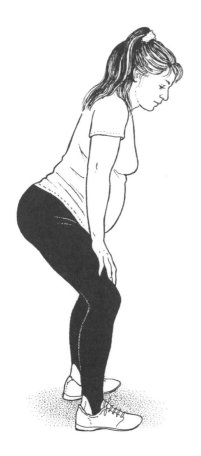

[B] Gently squeeze your butt and tilt your pelvis up so your butt lifts slightly off the floor and your pelvic bones shift toward your knees. Hold for two slow counts, then gently lower. Do 1–3 sets, 15–20 reps per set.

STANDING PELVIC TILT

Do the Pelvic Tilt in a standing position, leaning forward with your palms on your thighs.

TAILOR PRESS

Benefit: Strengthens your pelvic, hip, thigh, and core muscles.

[A] Sit on the floor with your knees bent and the soles of your feet pressed together. Grasp your ankles and pull your feet gently toward your body. Place your hands under your knees.

[B] While pressing your knees against your hands, press your hands up against your knees to create counterpressure. Hold for five slow counts, release for five counts. Do 1–3 sets, 5–10 reps per set.

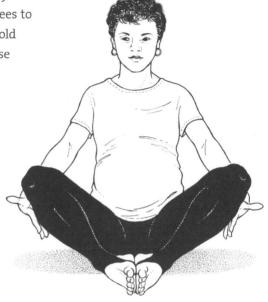

KEGELS

Benefit: Strengthens the pubococcygeal (PC) muscle, which controls the flow of urine.

[A] Stand, sit, or lie in any comfortable position.

[B] Contract the PC muscle as if you are stopping the flow of urine. Hold for 5 seconds, then relax for 5 seconds. Do Kegels twice a day, starting with 10 reps each time and gradually increasing to 100 or 4 sets of 25.

SQUAT

Benefit: Strengthens your butt, hips, and thighs.

[A] Stand with your feet hip-width apart with your hands on your hips or holding the back of a sturdy chair for support. Or, hold 3- to 5-pound weights with your arms at your sides.

[B] Bend your knees and squat down as far as you can. At the beginning of your pregnancy, you may be able to move until your thighs are parallel to the floor, but later you may be able to move only a few inches. Always move only to a point of comfort—never to the point of discomfort. Do 1–3 sets, 15–20 reps per set.

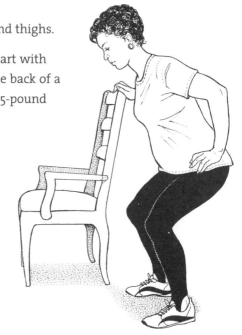

ROW

Benefit: Strengthens your upper/ mid back, shoulders, and biceps.

[A] Hold a 3- to 5-pound weight in your right hand and stand in front of a sturdy chair. Lean forward and place your left palm on the chair seat, and let your right arm hang straight down, palm facing in.

[B] Bend your right elbow to lift the weight up to waist height, then slowly lower it. Complete your reps, then switch arms. Do 1–3 sets, 15–20 reps per set.

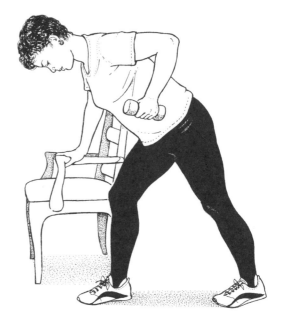

PUSH-UP

Benefit: Strengthens chest, shoulder, triceps, and core muscles.

[A] Position yourself face-down with your hands shoulder-distance apart, arms straight, and legs together, balancing on your palms and the underside of your toes. Pull your abs in to create a straight line from head to heels.

[B] Bend your elbows until your upper arms are parallel to floor, then press back up. Do 1–3 sets, 2–15 reps per set.

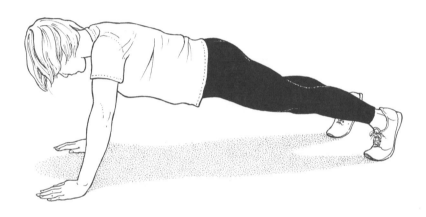

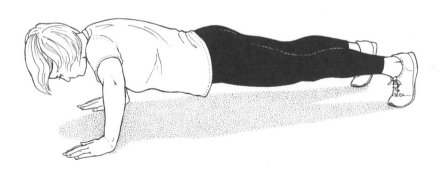

KNEELING PUSH-UP

Same as the Push-Up but balance on your thighs, just above your knees, with your palms placed flat on the floor.

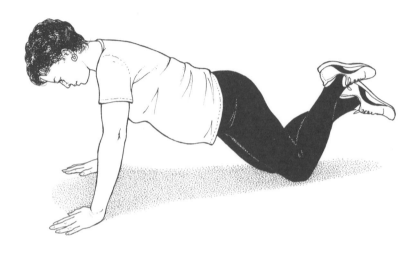

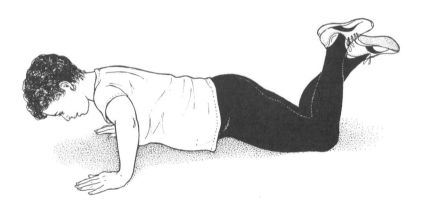

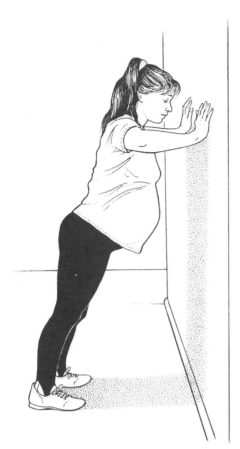

WALL PUSH-UP

Same as the Push-Up, but stand facing a wall, an arm's length away, with your hands pressed against the wall. Bend your arms to move your chest toward the wall.

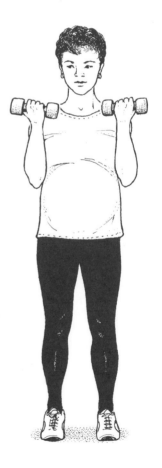

BICEPS CURL

Benefit: Strengthens your biceps.

[A] Sit, stand, or kneel with a 3- to 5-pound weight in each hand and your arms in front of your thighs, palms facing forward.

[B] Bend your elbows to curl the weights up to your shoulders, then lower the weights back down. Do 1–3 sets, 15–20 reps per set.

CHAIR DIP

Benefit: Strengthens your arm, chest, shoulder, and core muscles.

[A] Sit on the edge of a sturdy chair with your legs out straight, hands on either side, firmly grasping underside of chair seat. Slide your butt off the chair and straighten your arms so your weight is balanced on your palms and heels.

[B] Bend your elbows until your upper arms are close to parallel to floor, then press back up. Do 1–3 sets, 15–20 reps per set.

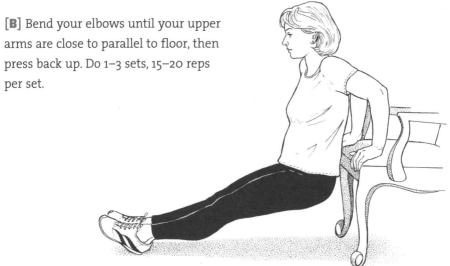

BENT-KNEE CHAIR DIP

Same as the Chair Dip, but with your knees bent and feet flat on floor.

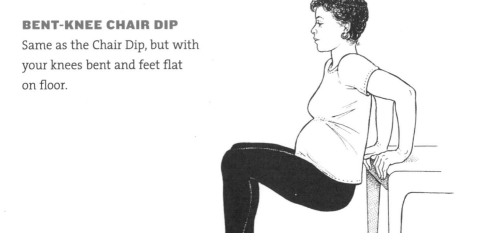

TREE POSE I

Benefit: Helps improve your balance.

[A] Stand tall with the sole of your right foot pressed against the inside of your upper left thigh, left knee pressed out to side. Hold your hands up in front of your chest in the prayer position.

[B] Hold the pose for up to 30 seconds. Repeat to the other side.

TREE POSE II

Same as the Tree Pose, but with the sole of your foot placed slightly lower, on the inside of the center of your thigh.

TREE POSE III

Same as the Tree Pose, but with the sole of your foot placed on the inside of your upper shin.

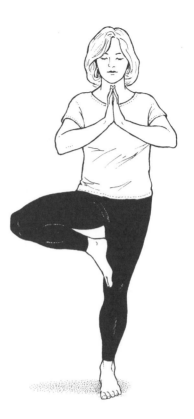

SIDE-LYING RELAXATION

Benefit: For rest and relaxation.

[A] Lie on either side with your head resting on your arm or on a pillow. Place a pillow or rolled-up towel between your thighs.

[B] Close your eyes and breathe deeply.

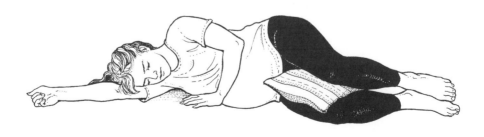

WHEN TO DO YOUR MUST-DO MOVES

EXERCISE	First Trimester	Second Trimester	Third Trimester
Crunchless Crunch	X		
Kneeling Crunchless Crunch		X	X
Pelvic Tilt	X		
Standing Pelvic Tilt		X	X
Tailor Press	X	X	X
Kegels	X	X	X
Squat	X	X	X
Row	X	X	X
Push-Up	X		
Kneeling Push-Up		X	
Wall Push-Up			X
Chair Dip	X		
Bent-Knee Chair Dip		X	X
Biceps Curl	X	X	X
Tree Pose I	X		
Tree Pose II		X	
Tree Pose III			X
Side-Lying Relaxation	X	X	X

WORKING AROUND YOUR PREGNANCY SYMPTOMS

Sure, the research says it's a good idea to exercise all the way through pregnancy, but how can you possibly lift a dumbbell when your wrists feel like they've been pounded with a hammer? How can you go for a power walk when your hips keep locking up and you have to stop every 4 minutes to pee? Or your feet are so swollen they look like loaves of bread?

Exercise during pregnancy isn't always a walk in the park, but in most cases, you can manage to work around even the most annoying symptoms. Below are tips to help you stay active even when you're big and uncomfortable.

These tips are meant to keep you moving throughout the nine months of pregnancy. They aren't intended as a substitute for medical advice, and you should check in with your medical team any time symptoms are severe. This list also isn't intended to cover more serious issues such as preeclampsia (pregnancy-induced high blood pressure in association with protein in the urine), fainting, blurred vision, vaginal bleeding, extreme swelling, or sharp belly pains. Warning: These could be signs of something more serious than morning sickness or an overzealous workout and should be checked out *immediately* by your healthcare provider.

SYMPTOM: MORNING SICKNESS

When you're feeling queasy, the last thing you want to do is sweat. But if you can push through those initial icky feelings, working out may actually help you feel better. Try eating a light, bland meal 30 minutes before your workout. Many women have good luck with plain crackers and ginger ale. Ginger, chamomile tea, lemons, and dry toast have also been known to quell the tummy flip-flops. Try taking your vitamins after, rather than before, your workout, and ask your healthcare provider about taking an antinausea medication—similar to antiseasickness meds—just before you exercise. Or, try wearing a soft cotton motion-sickness bracelet, available at most drugstores.

SYMPTOM: EXHAUSTION

Slow down your pace and/or break up your workout into several mini-sessions throughout the day rather than drag yourself through a 40-minute power walk. Or, alternate short spurts (1 to 5 minutes) of moderate-to-low intensity exercise with 1- to 2-minute rest breaks. Sometimes it's OK to bag your workout and take a nap instead. You'll be able to resume normal activity soon enough. Most women start to feel energized at some point during their pregnancy.

SYMPTOM: BIG BELLY

Try wearing a support belt to keep your bump from bouncing while you're on the move. Most large maternity-supply outlets carry them. Accept the fact that your belly may finally get so big in the last week or so that most workouts, even walking or weight training, will be too cumbersome to pull off. At this point, swimming and water aerobics are your best options. You may even want to simply float in the pool with a foam "noodle" under your knees and another one under your back.

SYMPTOM: ACHY WRISTS

At times, your hands and wrists may throb so much you can't practice the hand movements to "The Itsy Bitsy Spider." Numbness in your wrists, hands, and fingers, as well as tingling, burning, and outright pain, are quite common in the third trimester. The symptoms are due to fluid retention and swelling, which cause compression of the nerves in your forearms. To minimize these symptoms, hold your wrists straight when you lift weights or grasp the rails of a cardio machine, and place a towel underneath your palms for cushioning. Try icing your wrists 5 minutes or so before a workout.

SYMPTOM: SWOLLEN FEET

Swollen feet and ankles may become an issue at any stage of pregnancy but particularly the last few weeks. Your growing uterus puts pressure on the veins that return blood from your feet and legs, and changes in your blood chemistry also cause excess fluid to shift into your tissue. Fluid retention and dilated blood vessels may leave your entire body puffy, especially in the morning. If you have problems with swelling, use cold compresses on the affected areas. Using a footrest or lying down with your feet elevated may relieve ankle swelling. It may also help to swim, stand, or float in a pool. You'll probably want to avoid the treadmill and elliptical trainer, but consider the recumbent bike, which places much less pressure on your ankles. This is the time to lace up shoes that are at least half a size larger than normal; the extra wiggle room should help reduce the numbness that some women experience as the result of fat feet. Severe swelling should be checked out by your medical provider.

SYMPTOM: HIP AND BACK PAIN

As your body and uterus continue to expand, your posture may get thrown completely out of whack. In the presence of pregnancy hormones, your hips and lower spine move around more easily in preparation for birth, but this loosey-goosey pelvis also makes you more prone to hip and back pain. Try sleeping with a full-body support pillow between your legs, behind your back, or under your abdomen. You may need to sleep in a semireclined position rather than on one hip or the other.

Obviously, you should skip any workout that aggravates the pain. This may include certain exercises or excessive walking and bending. While most doctors recommend walking to keep in shape during pregnancy, for women with hip pain, this may be a problem. Some women are able to reduce aches with massage, physical therapy, chiropractic manipulation, yoga, or Pilates.

SYMPTOM: DEPRESSION OR MOOD SWINGS

Oh, those pesky pregnancy hormones! They're the reason you find yourself sobbing at *Everybody Loves Raymond* reruns or having a fit when your husband doesn't load the dishwasher correctly. Some women have the blues for weeks, while for others the sadness passes in a day or two. Exercise can definitely help lift your spirits and get you past the worst of it, but if you feel unbearably depressed for more than a day or two, be sure to tell your medical expert.

SYMPTOM: SHORTNESS OF BREATH

You may get winded easily as your uterus expands beneath your diaphragm, the muscle just below your lungs. The good news: this may improve when the baby settles deeper into your pelvis before delivery. In the meantime, practice good posture by standing up straight, centering your head between your shoulders, and relaxing your shoulders back and down. Try sleeping on your side rather than on your back so you don't hold your back in an overarched position for too long. Aerobic exercise can help relieve this feeling, as long as your healthcare provider says you're in the clear. By keeping your aerobic capacity pumped up, you'll have a greater capacity to suck in oxygen and to extract more of it from the air you breathe.

SYMPTOM: HEARTBURN

Before you got pregnant, you might have learned everything you knew about heartburn from watching Zantac commercials. Now? You feel like calling the fire department to douse the flames running wild in your chest—not exactly a joy when you're on the elliptical trainer. Pregnancy can bring on heartburn because the hormone progesterone relaxes the valve that separates your stomach and esophagus, allowing stomach acids to seep back up into the esophagus. The condition tends to worsen during the third trimester because your growing uterus crowds your stomach out of its normal position, further churning up stomach acids.

To keep that burning sensation and sour taste in check, eat small meals, drink plenty of fluids, and avoid spicy, greasy, and fatty foods. Ask your doctor if it's OK to take chewable antacids or stronger medications before you work out. You may need to try several medications before finding one that works for you.

SYMPTOM: SPIDER VEINS, VARICOSE VEINS, AND HEMORRHOIDS

Increased blood circulation may cause small reddish spots that sprout tiny blood vessels on your face, neck, upper chest, or arms, especially if you have fair skin. Varicose veins — blue or reddish lines beneath the surface of the skin — also may appear, particularly in your legs. Hemorrhoids, varicose veins in your rectum, are another highly unpleasant possibility. Spider veins may simply make you feel self-conscious in shorts, but hemorrhoids present a real problem during a workout. Bluntly put, it's hard to put your best foot forward when it feels like someone's placed shards of glass in your underwear. Try elevating your legs and wearing support stockings. Swimming may help, too, as it temporarily relieves some of the pressure in the affected areas. Be sure to include plenty of fiber in your diet and drink lots of fluids.

SYMPTOM: BURGEONING BREASTS

During your pregnancy you'll gain up to 3 pounds of breast tissue, and as delivery approaches, your nipples may start leaking colostrum, the yellowish fluid that will nourish your baby during the first few days of life. All this makes for a lot of extra bounce and chafe. Wear a sports bra that's a size larger than normal, and before you work out, coat your nipples liberally with a lubricant made for nipple protection.

SYMPTOM: FREQUENT URINATION

As your baby moves deeper into your pelvis, you'll feel more pressure on your bladder. You may find yourself getting most of your exercise by running to the bathroom. You may also leak urine when you work out and when you laugh, cough, or sneeze. If you experience these symptoms, plan your workouts so you're always close to a toilet. At the gym, choose the treadmill closest to the bathroom; plan your walking route in a neighborhood with a coffeehouse on every block, or locate the bathroom at a local park and do laps in the vicinity. Wear a pad in your workout clothes, so you'll have some protection if you drip a little. Watch for signs of a urinary-tract infection, such as urinating even more than usual, burning during urination, fever, abdominal pain, or backache. If you feel an infection coming on, check in with your practitioner.

WORKOUT GEAR CHECKLIST

Ten years ago, a pregnant exerciser had to make do with super-sized sweatpants and her partner's XXL undershirt, a look that was more "elephant draped in a tent" than *Fit Pregnancy* cover gal." Fortunately, these days there's no shortage of stylin', great-fitting maternity workout wear, from specially designed bike shorts and tennis skirts to moisture-wicking capris for yoga.

Since you're never quite sure when your growth spurts will hit or where exactly they're going to affect you most, it's best to buy items like pants, shorts, bras, and swimsuits as you go.

Here's a list of fitness gear you're likely to need as you stay active during your pregnancy.

➡ sneakers ½ to 1 size larger than normal

➡ 2 sports bras, one 1-cup-size larger and one 2-cup-sizes larger

➡ 2 pair maternity tights or shorts

➡ thin Lycra socks or hosiery (can help with swelling and circulation)

➡ 2 maternity workout tops

➡ maternity rain jacket

➡ water bottle

➡ snack pouch featuring emergency-contact window

➡ maternity support belt

➡ Vaseline or other lubricating gel to use during exercise for your extra-sensitive nipples and chafe points

➡ sunscreen

➡ hat

➡ maternity swimsuit

➡ specialized sports gear (tennis skirt, golf pants, yoga tights, cycling shorts for spinning bike)

➡ maternity workout DVDs

➡ place to list maternity workout class schedules

➡ stretch blocks (for when you can't lie on the floor anymore)

➡ exercise ball

➡ maternity briefs for active women

NUTRITION FOR THE NEXT NINE MONTHS

Before getting pregnant, you probably didn't obsess over your daily intake of folic acid or how many micrograms of iron your lunch supplied. Now? What you put in your mouth has probably become a focal point of your existence. If you're not busy worrying about whether a Starbucks caramel macchiato will harm the baby, you're thinking about how grossed out you are by the smell of refried beans or wondering whether you should be eating more protein.

There's no need to make yourself crazy, but these issues really are worth considering. The food choices you make while pregnant are probably more important than your eating habits at any other time in your life since they affect your baby's health as well as your own. Here are some key eating and nutritional strategies to follow for the next nine months.

➡ **Go easy on the extra calories.** Though you're eating for two, one of you is very tiny and not an excuse for the other one to become a Dunkin' Donuts frequent flyer. Research suggests that about 46 percent of pregnant women gain too much weight during pregnancy, increasing the risk of birth defects and gestational diabetes and possibly imprinting the baby to be predisposed to diabetes, heart disease, and obesity later in life. Also, when moms-to-be gain excess weight, they tend to retain extra poundage after pregnancy.

In the third trimester, you need about 300 extra calories per day per baby. That's a really small amount of food—one medium banana plus two tablespoons of peanut butter. It's also, incidentally, the number of calories in *one-third* of a Starbucks cinnamon scone—not the best way to spend your extra allotment. In the first trimester, doctors disagree on whether you need extra calories—if you're overweight, you likely don't—but rather than count calories, simply eat to appetite, and not more.

➡ **Manage your cravings and aversions.** You may resent any book that mentions trying to keep your cravings under control, and the truth is, for some women, even the mere suggestion of a healthier alternative than the salami-and-sour-cream wrap she craves will make her feel like ending her friendship with the person who is brave enough to bring it up. But do try to eat the healthiest foods you are able to. Most women don't experience weirdly decadent cravings throughout their pregnancy, so aim to get the bulk of your calories from nutritious foods, especially those rich in calcium, iron, folic acid, and other powerhouse nutrients. (For a list of those important vitamins and minerals and the best sources for them, see the Key Nutrient Needs During Pregnancy chart on page 32.) If you crave nonfoods such as charcoal, extremely burnt toast, cornstarch, clay, or chalk, tell your medical provider immediately, since this could signal a nutrient deficiency.

On the other hand, you may experience the mack daddy of all pregnancy symptoms: food aversions in the form of morning sickness. (And in case you haven't figured it out already, morning sickness can strike at any time throughout the day and at any point during your pregnancy.)

You can sometimes push through those initial icky feelings by eating something light and bland, like crackers or dry toast. Taking small sips of ginger ale or chamomile tea can help, or try a sports drink to replace fluids and electrolytes; this is important if you've been vomiting a lot. Another strategy: sucking on a hard candy or even a lemon. Wait to take your vitamins until bedtime. If you've been vomiting frequently, it's important to get that supplement down to help you meet your daily vitamin and mineral requirements.

➡ **Be a teetotaler.** For many years, the medical community vacillated about the safety of having an occasional drink during pregnancy, but there now seems to be a consensus: no amount of alcohol is safe to drink when you're with child. If you had a few glasses of wine before you realized you were pregnant, don't sweat it, but now that you know, skip the cocktails until after the baby is born.

Studies also suggest limiting caffeine, which is a bummer if you're having trouble trying to go cold turkey on your morning cup of joe when you're already feeling drained. Just try not to exceed 200 mg a day of caffeine (an 8-ounce cup of Starbucks coffee contains 250 mg). Recent research suggests that high caffeine consumption is linked to an increased risk of miscarriage, so stick within those limits or make the switch to decaf. (The Caffeine Counts chart on page 33 indicates the caffeine content of popular beverages.)

➡ **Fill up on fiber and fluids to help keep things moving.** Constipation is one of the more mysterious symptoms of pregnancy. You eat and eat and eat, but things rarely come out the other end. Thanks to hormones, iron supplements, and an intestine that gets scrunched into an ever-tighter space as the baby grows, you're going to feel pretty plugged up through much of your pregnancy.

The best anticonstipation strategy is eating 20 to 30 grams of fiber daily from veggies, fruits, and whole grains and downing plenty of fluids, at least 10 glasses a day, according to some experts. Sometimes nothing helps the problem, including doctor-sanctioned laxatives and stool softeners. However, you can't go wrong by increasing your fiber and fluid intake, since they're two habits that are healthy for both you and the baby.

➡ **Take your prenatal supplements faithfully.** A daily supplement will help you meet those pumped-up requirements for vitamins and minerals that are important for the baby's growth. Just be sure to have your medical team clear any other type of supplements you're taking. Supplements that never concerned you before may now be off-limits. For instance, you may be taking glucosamine for joint health, but there's not enough research on this substance to say whether it's safe for a developing fetus. Many herbal products and over-the-counter meds may be off limits, too.

➡ **Get your omega-3 fatty acids.** A diet rich in omega-3s can boost your baby's brain and neurological development before birth, likely leading to better vision, memory, and language comprehension in early childhood and can possibly reduce your risk of postpartum depression. Flaxseed oil, walnuts, and omega-3-fortified eggs are good sources of ALA, one of the three omega-3 fats, but fatty fish are the only reliable sources of the two more important omega-3s, EPA and DHA.

➡ **Avoid risky foods.** It's a myth that salt is the culprit behind preeclampsia, a form of high blood pressure in pregnant women, so feel free to shake a little extra onto your baked potato. Nevertheless, there are a number of foods that are a no-go during pregnancy.

Unpasteurized soft cheeses, such as Brie, Camembert, blue, and feta may harbor *Listeria monocytogenes* bacteria, which can lead to a dangerous form of food poisoning called listeriosis. Pregnant women are about 20 times more likely than everyone else to get listeriosis, which can cause miscarriage, premature delivery, stillbirth, and newborn infections. Hard, cooked, and processed cheeses are fine, as are cream cheese and cottage cheese.

This is also not the time to develop a sushi fixation, since raw or undercooked meat, poultry, seafood, and eggs are taboo for the duration. Unpasteurized milk and juice are also off limits. All of these foods can pass along foodborne illness.

Limit your consumption of fish high in mercury to no more than one 6-ounce serving once a week; these fish include shark, swordfish, fresh tuna (as opposed to canned tuna, which is fine), king mackerel, or tilefish. Super-high mercury consumption can be harmful to developing fetuses, but you can — and should — eat at least two weekly servings of fish that are low in mercury levels and high in omega-3 fatty acids. Good choices include shrimp, salmon (preferably wild), clams, sardines, and tilapia. You can find a complete list of the best and worst fish choices at www.oceansalive.org. The federal government also maintains a site on fish safety at www.epa.gov/waterscience/fishadvice/advice.html.

Other foods for your off-limits list: those that give you heartburn, that fiery sensation that starts in the pit of your stomach and travels upward into your throat. The usual suspects are carbonated drinks, caffeine, chocolate, acidic foods like citrus fruits and juices, tomatoes, mustard, vinegar, processed meats, mint products, and spicy, highly seasoned, fried, or fatty foods. In short — just about everything you love.

Nutrition experts have been divided in their advice to women about eating nuts and peanut butter during both pregnancy and breastfeeding. The consensus now seems to be that eating them won't cause your child to develop allergies.

KEY NUTRIENT NEEDS DURING PREGNANCY

NUTRIENT	NEEDED FOR	GOOD SOURCES
Protein	cell growth and blood production	lean meat, fish, poultry, egg whites, beans, tofu
Carbohydrate	daily energy production	breads, cereals, rice, potatoes, pasta, fruits, vegetables
Calcium	strong bones and teeth, muscle contraction, nerve function	milk, cheese, yogurt, sardines or salmon with bones, spinach
Iron	red blood cell production (needed to prevent anemia)	lean red meat, spinach, iron-fortified whole-grain breads and cereals
Vitamin A	healthy skin, good eyesight, growing bones	carrots, dark leafy greens, sweet potatoes
Vitamin C	healthy gums, teeth, and bones; assistance with iron absorption	citrus fruit, broccoli, tomatoes, fortified fruit juices
Vitamin B6	formation of red blood cells; effective use of protein, fat, and carbohydrates	pork, ham, whole-grain cereals, bananas
Vitamin B12*	formation of red blood cells, maintaining nervous system health	meat, fish, poultry, milk
Vitamin D	healthy bones and teeth; aids absorption of calcium	fortified milk, dairy products, cereals, and breads
Folic acid	blood and protein production, effective enzyme function	green leafy vegetables, dark yellow fruits and vegetables, beans, peas, nuts
Fat	body energy stores	avocado, nuts, peanut butter, vegetable oils
Zinc	preventing birth defects, premature delivery, and restricted fetal growth	meat, seafood, whole grains, legumes

*(Note: Vegetarians who don't eat dairy products need supplemental B12.)

CAFFEINE COUNTS

Experts recommend that pregnant women consume no more than 200 mg of caffeine a day. That eliminates a "tall" (12-ounce) coffee at Starbucks, which has 375 mg, but a latte? No problem. Here's a glance at the caffeine content of popular beverages.

	CAFFEINE (MG)*
Coffee, grande (16 oz.) Starbucks	550
Coffee, tall (12 oz.) Starbucks	375
Coffee, short (8 oz.) Starbucks	250
7-Eleven Big Gulp cola (64 oz.)	190
Maxwell House (8 oz.)	110
Caffe Americano, grande (16 oz.) Starbucks	105
Coffee, instant (8 oz.)	95**
Caffe Americano, tall (12 oz.) Starbucks	70
Caffe Latte or Cappuccino, grande (16 oz.) Starbucks	70
Caffe Mocha, grande (16 oz.) Starbucks	70
Espresso, double (2 oz.) Starbucks	70
Water, caffeinated (Edge 2 0), (8 oz.)	70
Cola (20 oz.)	60**
Mountain Dew (12 oz.)	55
Cola (16 oz.)	50**
Tea, leaf or bag (8 oz.)	50
Cola (12 oz.)	35**
Caffe Americano, short (8 oz.) Starbucks	35
Caffe Latte, short (8 oz.) or tall (12 oz.) Starbucks	35
Caffe Mocha, short (8 oz.) or tall (12 oz.) Starbucks	35
Cappuccino, short (8 oz.) or tall (12 oz.) Starbucks	35
Espresso (1 oz.) Starbucks	35
Tea, green or instant (8 oz.)	30**
Tea, bottles (12 oz.) or from instant mix (8 oz.)	14**
Coffee, decaf, grande (16 oz.) Starbucks	10
Coffee, decaf, short (8 oz.) or tall (12 oz.) Starbucks	10
Espresso, decaf (1 oz.) Starbucks	5
Coffee, decaf, nongourmet (8 oz.)	5**
Chocolate milk (1 oz.)	5**
Cocoa or hot chocolate (8 oz.)	5**
Tea, decaf (8 oz.)	0

* = Average caffeine levels for popular beverages, foods, and drugs (rounded to the nearest 5 milligrams)
** = Typical value

(*Source:* The Center for Science in the Public Interest, Nutrition Action Newsletter)

Daily Diary

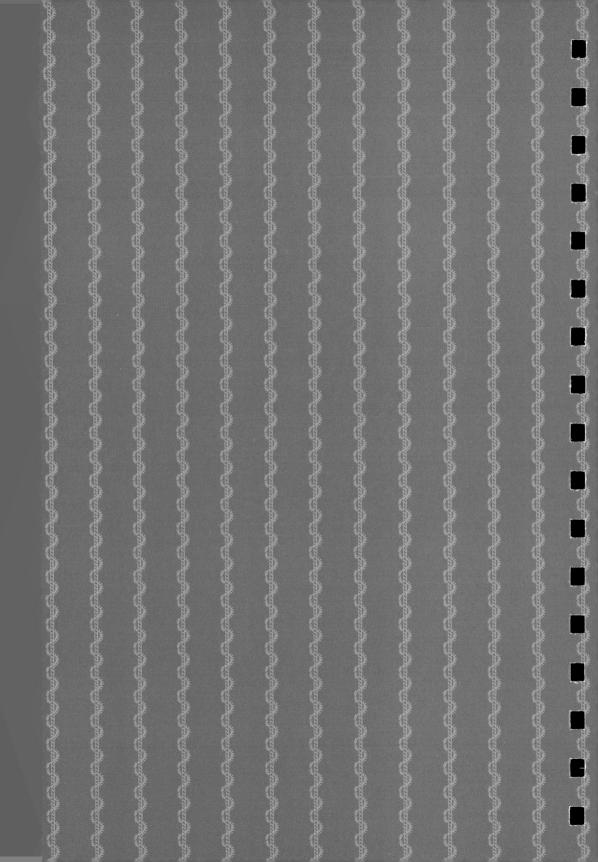

Filling In Your Log

Pregnancy may come with lots of rules — don't drink alcohol, take your supplements, don't kick your doctor in the face during an exam — but when it comes to filling out your daily log, you're welcome to do whatever the heck you want. How you use this log will depend, in part, on your personality. If you're a bookkeeper by nature or a fan of journaling, you'll probably scribble all over this diary, chronicling every last detail about your prenatal yoga classes and your cravings for tomatoes. If you're more of a minimalist, your log might simply note that you've done your Kegels and sum up the day in four words: "Ate falafel, threw up."

How much you record in your log also may depend on what stage of pregnancy you're in and how you're feeling. In the first trimester, you might be so wiped out that you can barely lift your pen to note that you swallowed your prenatal supplement. Two months later, you may gain all kinds of momentum from that pregnancy glow you've heard so much about but never really believed existed.

Following are suggestions for filling in each section of the log, but they're not the last word. Experiment and learn what works best for you.

GOALS FOR THE WEEK

When it comes to exercise goal-setting, pregnancy is unlike any other time in life: clearly, now isn't the time to shoot for a personal leg-press record or to beat your best 10k time. Still, it's a good idea to set some sort of objective for each week, whether you're striving to walk 30 minutes a day or drink milk with every meal. Setting goals will help you stay focused during times when you hardly have energy to lace up your walking shoes or when the size of your belly becomes inversely proportional to your motivation to move. Achieving your goals — and seeing the proof on paper — will give you a feeling of accomplishment, a sense that you've done something healthy each week for yourself and for your baby.

WEIGHT

Feel free to ignore the daily weight box. Some women—for the first time in their lives—like to track their weekly poundage. Others avert their eyes when they step on the scale at the doctor's office.

PRENATAL SUPPLEMENT

Sorry, this one you can't ignore—unless your doctor instructs you not to take a prenatal supplement. This may happen if the pills cause you to vomit constantly and you begin losing weight. Otherwise, check off this box daily.

KEGELS

Kegel exercises—described in detail on page 15—target your pelvic floor muscles, helping to strengthen your urethra, bladder, uterus, and rectum. Doing these exercises can give you extra oomph for childbirth and reduce your risk of postpartum incontinence. Ideally, you should do Kegels twice a day—hence the two Kegels boxes. In each box, record how many Kegels you did. Start with 10 twice a day, holding each for about 5 seconds, and aim to increase to 100 per day; you can break them up into shorter sets if 100 seems tedious. The Must-Do Strength Exercises section on page 13 explains why Kegels are key and how to do them.

EXERCISE

➡ Cardio: Describe your cardiovascular workout, whether you power walked, used the elliptical trainer, or took a prenatal water-aerobics class. In the gray boxes, note how long you exercised and your intensity level using the RPE method described on page 5.

➡ Strength: Use this space to record your muscle-toning workouts, such as Pilates, weight training, or core exercises done with a ball. If you lifted weights, you might note which muscle groups you targeted, such as "Abs, chest, back, arms." If you prefer to track your strength workouts in more detail, record the specific exercises, sets, and reps in the Daily Wrap-Up box.

Here's a first-trimester example:

Cardio elliptical
_____
Felt energized after!
_____
Intensity RPE 5–6
_____
Time 15 + 15 min., 5 min. rest in between
_____
Strength weight circuit, 12 reps per set, plus tree pose, pelvic tilts,
crunchless crunches
_____

Here's a third-trimester example:

Cardio Walked
_____
Slow, but still an accomplishment.
_____
Intensity 4–5
_____
Time 30 minutes
_____
Strength 2 sets: mini-squats, kegels, row, tree pose III
_____

RELAXATION

Did you meditate for 10 minutes this morning? Did you take a mellow pre-natal yoga class? Did you spend 15 minutes stretching at the gym? Here's the place to record these and other mind/body activities. Relaxation practices not only will help you chill out but will also help you hone some useful labor techniques.

NUTRITION

You can use this section in any number of ways. For example, you may want to track your food cravings; this can help you figure out if you've given into the urge to eat a 5-pound bag of M&Ms once too often. Tracking your aversions, meanwhile, can help you pinpoint just which culprits are making you toss your cookies. You could use this space to keep tabs on your fiber intake (if, for instance, you're suffering from constipation) or to track your caffeine consumption (if you worry you're too close to the 300 mg limit). Or, you can use this space to give yourself a pat on the back for choosing milk over soda at lunchtime.

Nutrition Woke up at 3 a.m. STARVING—ate cottage cheese
w/Triscuits; need to snack closer to bedtime.

Cravings Craving tomatoes like crazy. Tomato soup for lunch, pasta
w/marinara sauce for dinner.
Cereal w/yogurt at 10 p.m.

Aversions Suddenly grossed out by Mexican food! Beans and rice—blech!

MEDS/TESTS

Use this space to note when you have a doctor's appointment or a birthing class or a fitting for a nursing bra. If you're taking prescription medication — for example, daily progesterone shots following an in-vitro fertilization — this is the place to record your injections and any dosage changes prescribed by your doctor.

Meds / Tests Ultrasound, 8:30 a.m. We're having a girl!!!!

DAILY WRAP-UP

You can do just about anything with this box — note how many times you cried that day for no reason or document some odd new pigmentation that suddenly appeared on your face. Make notes about your energy level, your mood, your sex life, your varicose veins, your Dolly Parton–esque breasts, your insomnia, or your reaction when total strangers come up and rub your belly. Here is one place you're not likely to have writer's block!

DAILY WRAP-UP Wearing two sports bras—good idea; felt less bouncy
and a lot more athletic. Baby was kicking like crazy today!

WEEKLY WRAP-UP

This is the place to pause and reflect on the past seven days. Each week in pregnancy is a different adventure; there's always something new happening with your baby and your body, and you'll want to note the latest here.

➡ Goals: It's easy to set goals, but it's even easier to forget you ever did. This section keeps you honest, prompting you to look back at the goals you set the previous Monday and check off whether you met them. If you fell short, maybe you had unrealistic expectations. Or maybe pregnancy just intervened and nausea stopped you from exercising. That's OK! On the other hand, maybe you skipped your power walks just because you felt like watching a marathon of *Law & Order* reruns. In that case, get your butt moving, girl!

➡ Exercise: Add up your total cardio sessions, total cardio hours, and total strength. Make notes about how you're feeling in the exercise department. Is now the time to transition from jogging to walking or from walking to swimming? Are you feeling a surge of energy?

➡ Nutrition: What's the latest on the eating front? Have you gone completely mongo and eaten an entire birthday cake this week, or have you hurled your lunch virtually every day? This is a good place to note trends to share with your medical team.

➡ Reflections on the Week: Use this space to summarize the last seven Daily Wrap-Ups or to elaborate on topics you wrote about during the week.

40-WEEK DAILY DIARY

As you've probably deduced by now, the medical establishment calculates the length of pregnancy in an odd way: day 1 isn't actually the day of conception but rather the first day of your last menstrual period. So typically, by the time you've conceived, you're actually "two weeks" pregnant, and by the time you learn of your pregnancy, you're probably at least "four weeks" along—possibly further.

To keep things simple, this log tracks weeks the same way your health practitioner does, so skip the first two weeks, at least, and start tracking from the week you know that you're pregnant.

week 1

Dates: _____

Goals: _____
_____
_____

monday

WEIGHT [ ] **PRENATAL SUPPLEMENT** [ ] **KEGELS** [|]

EXERCISE

CARDIO: _____

RPE / HR: _____

_____

STRENGTH: _____

_____

_____

RELAXATION

NUTRITION

CRAVINGS: _____

AVERSIONS: _____

NOTES: _____

DAILY WRAP-UP

MEDS / TESTS

_____

_____

_____

_____

tuesday

WEIGHT [ ] **PRENATAL SUPPLEMENT** [ ] **KEGELS** [|]

EXERCISE

CARDIO: _____

RPE / HR: _____

_____

STRENGTH: _____

_____

_____

RELAXATION

NUTRITION

CRAVINGS: _____

AVERSIONS: _____

NOTES: _____

DAILY WRAP-UP

MEDS / TESTS

_____

_____

_____

_____

YOUR BABY THIS WEEK: Pregnancy math can be a little confusing, but here's how it works: although you're technically not pregnant for another two weeks, the official countdown begins on the first day of your last period.

wednesday

WEIGHT ☐ PRENATAL SUPPLEMENT ☐ KEGELS ☐☐

EXERCISE

CARDIO:

RPE / HR:

STRENGTH:

RELAXATION

DAILY WRAP-UP

NUTRITION

CRAVINGS:

AVERSIONS:

NOTES:

MEDS / TESTS

thursday

WEIGHT ☐ PRENATAL SUPPLEMENT ☐ KEGELS ☐☐

EXERCISE

CARDIO:

RPE / HR:

STRENGTH:

RELAXATION

DAILY WRAP-UP

NUTRITION

CRAVINGS:

AVERSIONS:

NOTES:

MEDS / TESTS

BY THE NUMBERS: **660 days:** Gestation period of the African elephant, the longest of any mammal. **450 days:** Gestation period of giraffes. **276 days:** Gestation of dolphins and chimpanzees. **266 days:** Gestation of humans. **12 days:** Gestation of opossums, the shortest for a mammal.

friday

WEIGHT ☐ PRENATAL SUPPLEMENT ☐ KEGELS ☐☐

EXERCISE _____

CARDIO: _____

RPE / HR: _____

_____

_____

STRENGTH: _____

_____

_____

RELAXATION

DAILY WRAP-UP

NUTRITION _____

CRAVINGS: _____

_____

AVERSIONS: _____

_____

NOTES: _____

_____

_____

MEDS / TESTS _____

_____

_____

_____

_____

saturday

WEIGHT ☐ PRENATAL SUPPLEMENT ☐ KEGELS ☐☐

EXERCISE _____

CARDIO: _____

RPE / HR: _____

_____

_____

STRENGTH: _____

_____

_____

RELAXATION

DAILY WRAP-UP

NUTRITION _____

CRAVINGS: _____

_____

AVERSIONS: _____

_____

NOTES: _____

_____

_____

MEDS / TESTS _____

_____

_____

_____

_____

"You should never say anything to a woman that even remotely suggests that you think she's pregnant unless you can see an actual baby emerging from her at that moment." — DAVE BARRY

sunday

WEIGHT [ ] PRENATAL SUPPLEMENT [ ] KEGELS [|]

EXERCISE

CARDIO: _____

RPE / HR: _____

_____

_____

STRENGTH: _____

_____

_____

RELAXATION

NUTRITION

CRAVINGS: _____

_____

AVERSIONS: _____

NOTES: _____

_____

_____

DAILY WRAP-UP

MEDS / TESTS

_____

_____

_____

_____

weekly wrap-up

GOALS   MET _____   EXCEEDED _____   MAYBE NEXT WEEK _____

EXERCISE   TOTAL CARDIO SESSIONS [ ]   TOTAL CARDIO HOURS [ ]   TOTAL STRENGTH SESSIONS [ ]

NOTES _____

_____

_____

NUTRITION

REFLECTIONS ON THE WEEK

week 2

Dates: _____

Goals: _____

_____

_____

monday

WEIGHT ☐   **PRENATAL SUPPLEMENT** ☐   KEGELS ☐☐

EXERCISE

CARDIO: _____

RPE / HR: _____

_____

_____

STRENGTH: _____

_____

_____

RELAXATION

NUTRITION

CRAVINGS: _____

AVERSIONS: _____

NOTES: _____

DAILY WRAP-UP

MEDS / TESTS

_____

_____

_____

tuesday

WEIGHT ☐   **PRENATAL SUPPLEMENT** ☐   KEGELS ☐☐

EXERCISE

CARDIO: _____

RPE / HR: _____

_____

_____

STRENGTH: _____

_____

_____

RELAXATION

NUTRITION

CRAVINGS: _____

AVERSIONS: _____

NOTES: _____

DAILY WRAP-UP

MEDS / TESTS

_____

_____

_____

_____

YOUR BABY THIS WEEK: Sperm and egg still haven't made their acquaintance, but the egg, with a lifespan of 12 to 24 hours, has started its journey down the fallopian tube. A few hundred sperm are heading its way; when the lead swimmer drills through the egg's shell, you've got yourself a baby!

wednesday

WEIGHT ☐   PRENATAL SUPPLEMENT ☐   KEGELS ☐☐

EXERCISE

CARDIO:

RPE / HR:

STRENGTH:

RELAXATION

NUTRITION

CRAVINGS:

AVERSIONS:

NOTES:

DAILY WRAP-UP

MEDS / TESTS

thursday

WEIGHT ☐   PRENATAL SUPPLEMENT ☐   KEGELS ☐☐

EXERCISE

CARDIO:

RPE / HR:

STRENGTH:

RELAXATION

NUTRITION

CRAVINGS:

AVERSIONS:

NOTES:

DAILY WRAP-UP

MEDS / TESTS

DID YOU KNOW? During pregnancy, the average woman's uterus expands up to 500 times its normal size, from the size of a peach to the size of a large beach ball. Blood volume increases up to 50 percent to meet the needs of the fetus and as a reserve against fluid loss that occurs during childbirth.

friday

WEIGHT ☐ PRENATAL SUPPLEMENT ☐ KEGELS ☐☐

EXERCISE

CARDIO:

RPE / HR:

STRENGTH:

RELAXATION

NUTRITION

CRAVINGS:

AVERSIONS:

NOTES:

DAILY WRAP-UP

MEDS / TESTS

saturday

WEIGHT ☐ PRENATAL SUPPLEMENT ☐ KEGELS ☐☐

EXERCISE

CARDIO:

RPE / HR:

STRENGTH:

RELAXATION

NUTRITION

CRAVINGS:

AVERSIONS:

NOTES:

DAILY WRAP-UP

MEDS / TESTS

THROUGH THE AGES: The first scientific pregnancy test, developed in 1928, involved injecting a woman's urine into mice. One hundred hours later, the mice were killed and their ovaries examined. A 1931 test with rabbits reduced the wait to 48 hours. The first home test, marketed in 1978, took 2 hours.

sunday

WEIGHT ☐ PRENATAL SUPPLEMENT ☐ KEGELS ☐ ☐

EXERCISE

CARDIO: _____

RPE / HR: _____

_____

_____

STRENGTH: _____

_____

RELAXATION

DAILY WRAP-UP

NUTRITION

CRAVINGS: _____

_____

AVERSIONS: _____

NOTES: _____

_____

_____

MEDS / TESTS

_____

_____

_____

_____

weekly wrap-up

GOALS   MET _____   EXCEEDED _____   MAYBE NEXT WEEK _____

EXERCISE   TOTAL CARDIO SESSIONS ☐   TOTAL CARDIO HOURS ☐   TOTAL STRENGTH SESSIONS ☐

NOTES _____

_____

_____

NUTRITION

REFLECTIONS ON THE WEEK

week

3

Dates:

Goals:

monday

WEIGHT | PRENATAL SUPPLEMENT | KEGELS

EXERCISE

CARDIO:

RPE / HR:

STRENGTH:

RELAXATION

NUTRITION

CRAVINGS:

AVERSIONS:

NOTES:

DAILY WRAP-UP

MEDS / TESTS

tuesday

WEIGHT | PRENATAL SUPPLEMENT | KEGELS

EXERCISE

CARDIO:

RPE / HR:

STRENGTH:

RELAXATION

NUTRITION

CRAVINGS:

AVERSIONS:

NOTES:

DAILY WRAP-UP

MEDS / TESTS

YOUR BABY THIS WEEK: As your burgeoning baby continues to cruise down the fallopian tube, its cells are dividing like crazy. Around midweek, the embryo, now a solid ball of about 200 cells, enters your uterus and floats around for a few days before finding a cozy spot to settle down.

wednesday

WEIGHT ☐   PRENATAL SUPPLEMENT ☐   KEGELS ☐☐

EXERCISE

CARDIO:

RPE / HR:

STRENGTH:

RELAXATION

NUTRITION

CRAVINGS:

AVERSIONS:

NOTES:

DAILY WRAP-UP

MEDS / TESTS

thursday

WEIGHT ☐   PRENATAL SUPPLEMENT ☐   KEGELS ☐☐

EXERCISE

CARDIO:

RPE / HR:

STRENGTH:

RELAXATION

NUTRITION

CRAVINGS:

AVERSIONS:

NOTES:

DAILY WRAP-UP

MEDS / TESTS

BY THE NUMBERS: 21.4: Average age of first-time mothers in the United States in 1970. **25.2:** Average age of first-time U.S. moms today. **27.7:** Average age of first-time mothers in Canada. **29.4:** Average age of first-time mothers in France. **30.4:** Average age of first-time mothers in Italy.

friday

WEIGHT ☐   PRENATAL SUPPLEMENT ☐   KEGELS ☐☐

EXERCISE

CARDIO:

RPE / HR:

STRENGTH:

RELAXATION

NUTRITION

CRAVINGS:

AVERSIONS:

NOTES:

MEDS / TESTS

DAILY WRAP-UP

saturday

WEIGHT ☐   PRENATAL SUPPLEMENT ☐   KEGELS ☐☐

EXERCISE

CARDIO:

RPE / HR:

STRENGTH:

RELAXATION

NUTRITION

CRAVINGS:

AVERSIONS:

NOTES:

MEDS / TESTS

DAILY WRAP-UP

> "There is one other little thing about telling your father you are pregnant: this may be the very first time in your entire life that you have boldly declared to him that you are no longer a virgin."
> — VICKI IOVINE, The Girlfriends' Guide to Pregnancy

sunday

WEIGHT ☐ PRENATAL SUPPLEMENT ☐ KEGELS ☐☐

EXERCISE

CARDIO: _____

RPE / HR: _____

_____

_____

STRENGTH: _____

_____

_____

RELAXATION

NUTRITION

CRAVINGS: _____

AVERSIONS: _____

NOTES: _____

_____

_____

MEDS / TESTS

_____

_____

_____

_____

DAILY WRAP-UP

weekly wrap-up

GOALS   MET _____   EXCEEDED _____   MAYBE NEXT WEEK _____

EXERCISE   TOTAL CARDIO SESSIONS ☐   TOTAL CARDIO HOURS ☐   TOTAL STRENGTH SESSIONS ☐

NOTES _____

_____

_____

NUTRITION

REFLECTIONS ON THE WEEK

week 4

Dates: _____

Goals: _____
_____
_____

monday

WEIGHT [ ] **PRENATAL SUPPLEMENT** [ ] **KEGELS** [ ][ ]

EXERCISE
CARDIO: _____
RPE / HR: _____
_____
_____
STRENGTH: _____
_____
_____

RELAXATION

DAILY WRAP-UP

NUTRITION
CRAVINGS: _____
_____
AVERSIONS: _____
_____
NOTES: _____
_____

MEDS / TESTS
_____
_____
_____
_____

tuesday

WEIGHT [ ] **PRENATAL SUPPLEMENT** [ ] **KEGELS** [ ][ ]

EXERCISE
CARDIO: _____
RPE / HR: _____
_____
_____
STRENGTH: _____
_____
_____

RELAXATION

DAILY WRAP-UP

NUTRITION
CRAVINGS: _____
_____
AVERSIONS: _____
_____
NOTES: _____
_____

MEDS / TESTS
_____
_____
_____
_____

YOUR BABY THIS WEEK: Implantation is a done deal, and the placenta has formed, tapping in to your circulation. It's the placenta that produces hCG, the hormone detected by pregnancy tests. A sensitive home test can indicate pregnancy as soon as day 10 after fertilization.

wednesday

WEIGHT ☐ PRENATAL SUPPLEMENT ☐ KEGELS ☐ ☐

EXERCISE

CARDIO:

RPE / HR:

STRENGTH:

RELAXATION

DAILY WRAP-UP

NUTRITION

CRAVINGS:

AVERSIONS:

NOTES:

MEDS / TESTS

thursday

WEIGHT ☐ PRENATAL SUPPLEMENT ☐ KEGELS ☐ ☐

EXERCISE

CARDIO:

RPE / HR:

STRENGTH:

RELAXATION

DAILY WRAP-UP

NUTRITION

CRAVINGS:

AVERSIONS:

NOTES:

MEDS / TESTS

DID YOU KNOW? Dad decides what gender your baby will be. When a baby is conceived, it gets one sex chromosome from each parent. From Mom — who's an XX — baby always gets an X chromosome. From Dad, baby gets either an X or a Y.

friday

WEIGHT ☐ PRENATAL SUPPLEMENT ☐ KEGELS ☐☐

EXERCISE

CARDIO:

RPE / HR:

STRENGTH:

RELAXATION

DAILY WRAP-UP

NUTRITION

CRAVINGS:

AVERSIONS:

NOTES:

MEDS / TESTS

saturday

WEIGHT ☐ PRENATAL SUPPLEMENT ☐ KEGELS ☐☐

EXERCISE

CARDIO:

RPE / HR:

STRENGTH:

RELAXATION

DAILY WRAP-UP

NUTRITION

CRAVINGS:

AVERSIONS:

NOTES:

MEDS / TESTS

THROUGH THE AGES: Seventeenth-century doctors believed babies were completely developed at conception and during gestation simply grew. Some claimed these mini-humans were housed in sperm heads and were visible under a microscope. Other believed the tiny, fully formed babies were lodged in the eggs.

sunday

WEIGHT ☐ PRENATAL SUPPLEMENT ☐ KEGELS ☐☐

EXERCISE

CARDIO:

RPE / HR:

STRENGTH:

RELAXATION

DAILY WRAP-UP

NUTRITION

CRAVINGS:

AVERSIONS:

NOTES:

MEDS / TESTS

weekly wrap-up

GOALS   MET _____   EXCEEDED _____   MAYBE NEXT WEEK _____

EXERCISE   TOTAL CARDIO SESSIONS ☐   TOTAL CARDIO HOURS ☐   TOTAL STRENGTH SESSIONS ☐

NOTES

NUTRITION

REFLECTIONS ON THE WEEK

week

5

Dates: _____

Goals: _____
_____
_____
_____

monday

WEIGHT [ ]   **PRENATAL SUPPLEMENT** [ ]   **KEGELS** [ ][ ]

EXERCISE _____

CARDIO: _____

RPE / HR: _____

_____

_____

STRENGTH: _____

_____

_____

RELAXATION

NUTRITION _____

CRAVINGS: _____

_____

AVERSIONS: _____

_____

NOTES: _____

_____

DAILY WRAP-UP

MEDS / TESTS

_____

_____

_____

_____

tuesday

WEIGHT [ ]   **PRENATAL SUPPLEMENT** [ ]   **KEGELS** [ ][ ]

EXERCISE _____

CARDIO: _____

RPE / HR: _____

_____

_____

STRENGTH: _____

_____

_____

RELAXATION

NUTRITION _____

CRAVINGS: _____

_____

AVERSIONS: _____

_____

NOTES: _____

_____

DAILY WRAP-UP

MEDS / TESTS

_____

_____

_____

_____

YOUR BABY THIS WEEK: A busy week for baby: the creation of the skeleton, eyes, and ears are in full swing, and her brain has divided into two lobes. Baby's heart has begun to drum a steady beat, though the sound is too faint to hear on ultrasound. Baby measures about one-eighth of an inch, the size of a sesame seed.

wednesday

WEIGHT ☐   PRENATAL SUPPLEMENT ☐   KEGELS ☐☐

EXERCISE

CARDIO:

RPE / HR:

STRENGTH:

RELAXATION

NUTRITION

CRAVINGS:

AVERSIONS:

NOTES:

DAILY WRAP-UP

MEDS / TESTS

thursday

WEIGHT ☐   PRENATAL SUPPLEMENT ☐   KEGELS ☐☐

EXERCISE

CARDIO:

RPE / HR:

STRENGTH:

RELAXATION

NUTRITION

CRAVINGS:

AVERSIONS:

NOTES:

DAILY WRAP-UP

MEDS / TESTS

BY THE NUMBERS: **65:** Percent of women who report feeling some degree of sickness early in pregnancy. **5:** Percent of women who experience nausea until term. **33:** Percent who suffer a strong aversion to animal products, particularly meat, fish, and eggs.

friday

WEIGHT [ ] PRENATAL SUPPLEMENT [ ] KEGELS [ ][ ]

EXERCISE

CARDIO:

RPE / HR:

STRENGTH:

RELAXATION

NUTRITION

CRAVINGS:

AVERSIONS:

NOTES:

DAILY WRAP-UP

MEDS / TESTS

saturday

WEIGHT [ ] PRENATAL SUPPLEMENT [ ] KEGELS [ ][ ]

EXERCISE

CARDIO:

RPE / HR:

STRENGTH:

RELAXATION

NUTRITION

CRAVINGS:

AVERSIONS:

NOTES:

DAILY WRAP-UP

MEDS / TESTS

"I'm like, oh my God, can you believe it just happened?"
— **CHRISTINA AGUILERA,** on getting pregnant while still on tour

sunday

WEIGHT PRENATAL SUPPLEMENT KEGELS

EXERCISE

CARDIO:

RPE / HR:

STRENGTH:

RELAXATION

NUTRITION

CRAVINGS:

AVERSIONS:

NOTES:

DAILY WRAP-UP

MEDS / TESTS

weekly wrap-up

GOALS   MET _____   EXCEEDED _____   MAYBE NEXT WEEK _____

EXERCISE   TOTAL CARDIO SESSIONS   TOTAL CARDIO HOURS   TOTAL STRENGTH SESSIONS

NOTES

NUTRITION

REFLECTIONS ON THE WEEK

week 6

Dates: _____

Goals: _____

_____

_____

monday

WEIGHT ☐ PRENATAL SUPPLEMENT ☐ KEGELS ☐☐

EXERCISE

CARDIO: _____

RPE / HR: _____

_____

_____

STRENGTH: _____

_____

_____

RELAXATION

DAILY WRAP-UP

NUTRITION

CRAVINGS: _____

AVERSIONS: _____

NOTES: _____

MEDS / TESTS

_____

_____

_____

_____

tuesday

WEIGHT ☐ PRENATAL SUPPLEMENT ☐ KEGELS ☐☐

EXERCISE

CARDIO: _____

RPE / HR: _____

_____

_____

STRENGTH: _____

_____

_____

RELAXATION

DAILY WRAP-UP

NUTRITION

CRAVINGS: _____

AVERSIONS: _____

NOTES: _____

MEDS / TESTS

_____

_____

_____

_____

YOUR BABY THIS WEEK: If you're beginning to feel more attached to your baby, maybe it's because the umbilical cord has begun to form. Baby's limb buds have sprouted tiny webbed structures that will someday be your little muffin's fingers and toes. Baby's jaws and eyelids are developing, too.

wednesday

WEIGHT ☐   PRENATAL SUPPLEMENT ☐   KEGELS ☐☐

EXERCISE

CARDIO:

RPE / HR:

STRENGTH:

RELAXATION

NUTRITION

CRAVINGS:

AVERSIONS:

NOTES:

DAILY WRAP-UP

MEDS / TESTS

thursday

WEIGHT ☐   PRENATAL SUPPLEMENT ☐   KEGELS ☐☐

EXERCISE

CARDIO:

RPE / HR:

STRENGTH:

RELAXATION

NUTRITION

CRAVINGS:

AVERSIONS:

NOTES:

DAILY WRAP-UP

MEDS / TESTS

DID YOU KNOW? Almost all of the developments that a human baby will experience in its first year — advances in cognition, motor skills, and vision — have already taken place in a baby chimpanzee before it is born.

friday

WEIGHT ☐ PRENATAL SUPPLEMENT ☐ KEGELS ☐☐

EXERCISE

CARDIO:

RPE / HR:

STRENGTH:

RELAXATION

NUTRITION

CRAVINGS:

AVERSIONS:

NOTES:

DAILY WRAP-UP

MEDS / TESTS

saturday

WEIGHT ☐ PRENATAL SUPPLEMENT ☐ KEGELS ☐☐

EXERCISE

CARDIO:

RPE / HR:

STRENGTH:

RELAXATION

NUTRITION

CRAVINGS:

AVERSIONS:

NOTES:

DAILY WRAP-UP

MEDS / TESTS

THROUGH THE AGES: It was a nineteenth-century German obstetrician named Naegele who decreed that pregnancy should last 10 lunar months — 40 weeks — even though a woman is actually pregnant for only 38 weeks. Naegele used the first day of the woman's last period as day 1.

sunday

WEIGHT ☐ PRENATAL SUPPLEMENT ☐ KEGELS ☐☐

EXERCISE

CARDIO: _____

RPE / HR: _____

_____

_____

STRENGTH: _____

_____

_____

RELAXATION

NUTRITION

CRAVINGS: _____

_____

AVERSIONS: _____

_____

NOTES: _____

DAILY WRAP-UP

MEDS / TESTS

_____

_____

_____

_____

_____

weekly wrap-up

GOALS   MET _____   EXCEEDED _____   MAYBE NEXT WEEK _____

EXERCISE   TOTAL CARDIO SESSIONS ☐   TOTAL CARDIO HOURS ☐   TOTAL STRENGTH SESSIONS ☐

NOTES _____

_____

_____

NUTRITION

REFLECTIONS ON THE WEEK

week 7

Dates: _____

Goals: _____

_____

_____

monday

| WEIGHT | | PRENATAL SUPPLEMENT | | KEGELS | |

EXERCISE

CARDIO: _____

RPE / HR: _____

_____

_____

STRENGTH: _____

_____

_____

RELAXATION

DAILY WRAP-UP

NUTRITION

CRAVINGS: _____

AVERSIONS: _____

NOTES: _____

MEDS / TESTS

_____

_____

_____

_____

tuesday

| WEIGHT | | PRENATAL SUPPLEMENT | | KEGELS | |

EXERCISE

CARDIO: _____

RPE / HR: _____

_____

_____

STRENGTH: _____

_____

RELAXATION

DAILY WRAP-UP

NUTRITION

CRAVINGS: _____

AVERSIONS: _____

NOTES: _____

MEDS / TESTS

_____

_____

_____

_____

YOUR BABY THIS WEEK: Baby has a tongue, kidneys, flipper-like arms, and legs that look like paddles. The big story: baby's brain is growing at record speed, with nerve cells forming at a rate of 100,000 per minute. By the end of the week, baby is about half an inch long, the size of a caterpillar.

wednesday

WEIGHT ☐   PRENATAL SUPPLEMENT ☐   KEGELS ☐☐

EXERCISE

CARDIO:

RPE / HR:

STRENGTH:

RELAXATION

NUTRITION

CRAVINGS:

AVERSIONS:

NOTES:

MEDS / TESTS

DAILY WRAP-UP

thursday

WEIGHT ☐   PRENATAL SUPPLEMENT ☐   KEGELS ☐☐

EXERCISE

CARDIO:

RPE / HR:

STRENGTH:

RELAXATION

NUTRITION

CRAVINGS:

AVERSIONS:

NOTES:

MEDS / TESTS

DAILY WRAP-UP

friday

WEIGHT ☐ PRENATAL SUPPLEMENT ☐ KEGELS ☐☐

EXERCISE

CARDIO:

RPE / HR:

STRENGTH:

RELAXATION

NUTRITION

CRAVINGS:

AVERSIONS:

NOTES:

MEDS / TESTS

DAILY WRAP-UP

saturday

WEIGHT ☐ PRENATAL SUPPLEMENT ☐ KEGELS ☐☐

EXERCISE

CARDIO:

RPE / HR:

STRENGTH:

RELAXATION

NUTRITION

CRAVINGS:

AVERSIONS:

NOTES:

MEDS / TESTS

DAILY WRAP-UP

> "When you're pregnant you don't need a song to come on the radio to make you cry. You just need to hear a traffic report and the floodgates will open."
> — JENNY MCCARTHY, in Belly Laughs

sunday

WEIGHT [   ] PRENATAL SUPPLEMENT [   ] KEGELS [   ][   ]

EXERCISE

CARDIO: _____

RPE / HR: _____

_____

_____

STRENGTH: _____

_____

_____

RELAXATION

NUTRITION

CRAVINGS: _____

AVERSIONS: _____

NOTES: _____

_____

DAILY WRAP-UP

MEDS / TESTS

_____

_____

_____

_____

weekly wrap-up

GOALS   MET _____   EXCEEDED _____   MAYBE NEXT WEEK _____

EXERCISE   TOTAL CARDIO SESSIONS [   ]   TOTAL CARDIO HOURS [   ]   TOTAL STRENGTH SESSIONS [   ]

NOTES _____

_____

_____

NUTRITION

REFLECTIONS ON THE WEEK

week 8

Dates:

Goals:

monday

WEIGHT | **PRENATAL SUPPLEMENT** | **KEGELS**

EXERCISE

CARDIO:

RPE / HR:

STRENGTH:

RELAXATION

NUTRITION

CRAVINGS:

AVERSIONS:

NOTES:

DAILY WRAP-UP

MEDS / TESTS

tuesday

WEIGHT | **PRENATAL SUPPLEMENT** | **KEGELS**

EXERCISE

CARDIO:

RPE / HR:

STRENGTH:

RELAXATION

NUTRITION

CRAVINGS:

AVERSIONS:

NOTES:

DAILY WRAP-UP

MEDS / TESTS

YOUR BABY THIS WEEK: With earlobes, visible elbow and knee joints, a four-chambered heart, and most major organs developing, baby is starting to resemble a mini-person! Baby may take his newfound sense of touch for a test drive by stroking his face, sucking a thumb, or stretching out his body.

wednesday

WEIGHT ☐ PRENATAL SUPPLEMENT ☐ KEGELS ☐☐

EXERCISE
CARDIO:
RPE / HR:

STRENGTH:

RELAXATION

NUTRITION
CRAVINGS:

AVERSIONS:

NOTES:

DAILY WRAP-UP

MEDS / TESTS

thursday

WEIGHT ☐ PRENATAL SUPPLEMENT ☐ KEGELS ☐☐

EXERCISE
CARDIO:
RPE / HR:

STRENGTH:

RELAXATION

NUTRITION
CRAVINGS:

AVERSIONS:

NOTES:

DAILY WRAP-UP

MEDS / TESTS

DID YOU KNOW? About 25 percent of expectant dads develop couvade syndrome, experiencing many of the same physical symptoms, such as stomachaches, weight gain, and bloating, that their pregnant partners have. Couvade is a French word meaning "to hatch."

friday

WEIGHT ☐ PRENATAL SUPPLEMENT ☐ KEGELS ☐☐

EXERCISE

CARDIO:

RPE / HR:

STRENGTH:

RELAXATION

NUTRITION

CRAVINGS:

AVERSIONS:

NOTES:

MEDS / TESTS

DAILY WRAP-UP

saturday

WEIGHT ☐ PRENATAL SUPPLEMENT ☐ KEGELS ☐☐

EXERCISE

CARDIO:

RPE / HR:

STRENGTH:

RELAXATION

NUTRITION

CRAVINGS:

AVERSIONS:

NOTES:

MEDS / TESTS

DAILY WRAP-UP

THROUGH THE AGES: When Lucille Ball's real-life pregnancy was written into I Love Lucy in 1952, it was the first time a TV character had been portrayed as pregnant. CBS hired three clergymen to oversee each script. The show aired at a time when married couples on TV slept in separate beds.

sunday

WEIGHT ☐ PRENATAL SUPPLEMENT ☐ KEGELS ☐☐

EXERCISE

CARDIO:

RPE / HR:

STRENGTH:

RELAXATION

NUTRITION

CRAVINGS:

AVERSIONS:

NOTES:

DAILY WRAP-UP

MEDS / TESTS

weekly wrap-up

GOALS MET _____ EXCEEDED _____ MAYBE NEXT WEEK _____

EXERCISE TOTAL CARDIO SESSIONS ☐ TOTAL CARDIO HOURS ☐ TOTAL STRENGTH SESSIONS ☐

NOTES

NUTRITION

REFLECTIONS ON THE WEEK

week 9

Dates: _____

Goals: _____
_____
_____

monday

WEIGHT [ ]   **PRENATAL SUPPLEMENT** [ ]   **KEGELS** [ ][ ]

EXERCISE

CARDIO:

RPE / HR:
_____
_____

STRENGTH:
_____
_____

RELAXATION

NUTRITION

CRAVINGS:
_____

AVERSIONS:
_____

NOTES:
_____
_____

DAILY WRAP-UP

MEDS / TESTS
_____
_____
_____
_____

tuesday

WEIGHT [ ]   **PRENATAL SUPPLEMENT** [ ]   **KEGELS** [ ][ ]

EXERCISE

CARDIO:

RPE / HR:
_____
_____

STRENGTH:
_____
_____

RELAXATION

NUTRITION

CRAVINGS:
_____

AVERSIONS:
_____

NOTES:
_____
_____

DAILY WRAP-UP

MEDS / TESTS
_____
_____
_____
_____

YOUR BABY THIS WEEK: How big is baby now? About the size of a grape. But this little grape has eyelids, tiny webbed fingers, the beginnings of vertebral discs, and arms that are starting to bend at the elbow. Baby also has a reflex response to touch; if an object touches her head, baby will turn away.

wednesday

WEIGHT | PRENATAL SUPPLEMENT | KEGELS

EXERCISE

CARDIO:

RPE / HR:

STRENGTH:

RELAXATION

NUTRITION

CRAVINGS:

AVERSIONS:

NOTES:

DAILY WRAP-UP

MEDS / TESTS

thursday

WEIGHT | PRENATAL SUPPLEMENT | KEGELS

EXERCISE

CARDIO:

RPE / HR:

STRENGTH:

RELAXATION

NUTRITION

CRAVINGS:

AVERSIONS:

NOTES:

DAILY WRAP-UP

MEDS / TESTS

BY THE NUMBERS: **30:** Typical number of pounds women gain during pregnancy. **7.5:** Average weight, in pounds, of a newborn. **8:** Pounds of extra blood and body fluids. **7:** Pounds of extra fat stored. **5.5:** Pounds accounting for uterine growth, placenta, and amniotic fluid. **2:** Pounds of breast growth.

friday

WEIGHT ☐ PRENATAL SUPPLEMENT ☐ KEGELS ☐☐

EXERCISE _____

CARDIO: _____

RPE / HR: _____

_____

_____

STRENGTH: _____

_____

_____

RELAXATION

NUTRITION _____

CRAVINGS: _____

_____

AVERSIONS: _____

_____

NOTES: _____

_____

DAILY WRAP-UP

MEDS / TESTS

_____

_____

_____

_____

_____

saturday

WEIGHT ☐ PRENATAL SUPPLEMENT ☐ KEGELS ☐☐

EXERCISE _____

CARDIO: _____

RPE / HR: _____

_____

_____

STRENGTH: _____

_____

_____

RELAXATION

NUTRITION _____

CRAVINGS: _____

_____

AVERSIONS: _____

_____

NOTES: _____

_____

DAILY WRAP-UP

MEDS / TESTS

_____

_____

_____

_____

_____

"I'm convinced the doctor who coined the phrase 'morning sickness' was trying to trick women into thinking they'd feel better by the afternoon — and to trick their husbands into thinking they'd be safe by evening."
—IAN DAVIS, author of My Boys Can Swim

sunday

WEIGHT ☐   PRENATAL SUPPLEMENT ☐   KEGELS ☐ ☐

EXERCISE

CARDIO:

RPE / HR:

STRENGTH:

RELAXATION

NUTRITION

CRAVINGS:

AVERSIONS:

NOTES:

DAILY WRAP-UP

MEDS / TESTS

weekly wrap-up

GOALS   MET _____   EXCEEDED _____   MAYBE NEXT WEEK _____

EXERCISE   TOTAL CARDIO SESSIONS ☐   TOTAL CARDIO HOURS ☐   TOTAL STRENGTH SESSIONS ☐

NOTES

NUTRITION

REFLECTIONS ON THE WEEK

week 10

Dates: _____

Goals: _____
_____
_____

monday

WEIGHT ☐ PRENATAL SUPPLEMENT ☐ KEGELS ☐☐

EXERCISE

CARDIO: _____

RPE / HR: _____

_____

_____

STRENGTH: _____

_____

_____

RELAXATION

DAILY WRAP-UP

NUTRITION

CRAVINGS: _____

AVERSIONS: _____

NOTES: _____

_____

MEDS / TESTS

_____

_____

_____

_____

tuesday

WEIGHT ☐ PRENATAL SUPPLEMENT ☐ KEGELS ☐☐

EXERCISE

CARDIO: _____

RPE / HR: _____

_____

_____

STRENGTH: _____

_____

_____

RELAXATION

DAILY WRAP-UP

NUTRITION

CRAVINGS: _____

AVERSIONS: _____

NOTES: _____

_____

MEDS / TESTS

_____

_____

_____

_____

YOUR BABY THIS WEEK: Finally! Baby is hefty enough for your practitioner to estimate his weight — probably around a quarter ounce. In other developments, baby now has an upper lip, external ears, separated fingers and toes, and the beginnings of taste buds.

wednesday

WEIGHT ☐ PRENATAL SUPPLEMENT ☐ KEGELS ☐☐

EXERCISE

CARDIO:

RPE / HR:

STRENGTH:

RELAXATION

NUTRITION

CRAVINGS:

AVERSIONS:

NOTES:

DAILY WRAP-UP

MEDS / TESTS

thursday

WEIGHT ☐ PRENATAL SUPPLEMENT ☐ KEGELS ☐☐

EXERCISE

CARDIO:

RPE / HR:

STRENGTH:

RELAXATION

NUTRITION

CRAVINGS:

AVERSIONS:

NOTES:

DAILY WRAP-UP

MEDS / TESTS

DID YOU KNOW? Whether your baby is a lefty or a righty is determined as early as 10 weeks into your pregnancy. Babies in the womb favor one hand over the other, and it's the same one they'll prefer in life.

friday

WEIGHT ☐ | PRENATAL SUPPLEMENT ☐ | KEGELS ☐☐

EXERCISE

CARDIO:

RPE / HR:

STRENGTH:

RELAXATION

NUTRITION

CRAVINGS:

AVERSIONS:

NOTES:

DAILY WRAP-UP

MEDS / TESTS

saturday

WEIGHT ☐ | PRENATAL SUPPLEMENT ☐ | KEGELS ☐☐

EXERCISE

CARDIO:

RPE / HR:

STRENGTH:

RELAXATION

NUTRITION

CRAVINGS:

AVERSIONS:

NOTES:

DAILY WRAP-UP

MEDS / TESTS

THROUGH THE AGES: In ancient Chinese tradition, anything that affects a woman's mind also affects her unborn child. To ensure her baby will be talented and beautiful, a pregnant woman must not gossip or lose her temper but instead should read lovely stories and poetry and listen to fine music.

sunday

WEIGHT ☐

PRENATAL SUPPLEMENT ☐

KEGELS ☐ ☐

EXERCISE

CARDIO: _____

RPE / HR: _____

_____

_____

STRENGTH: _____

_____

RELAXATION

NUTRITION

CRAVINGS: _____

_____

AVERSIONS: _____

_____

NOTES: _____

_____

DAILY WRAP-UP

MEDS / TESTS

_____

_____

_____

_____

weekly wrap-up

GOALS   MET _____   EXCEEDED _____   MAYBE NEXT WEEK _____

EXERCISE   TOTAL CARDIO SESSIONS ☐   TOTAL CARDIO HOURS ☐   TOTAL STRENGTH SESSIONS ☐

NOTES _____

_____

_____

NUTRITION

REFLECTIONS ON THE WEEK

week 11

Dates: _____

Goals: _____
_____
_____

monday

WEIGHT ☐ PRENATAL SUPPLEMENT ☐ KEGELS ☐☐

EXERCISE

CARDIO: _____

RPE / HR: _____

_____

STRENGTH: _____

_____

_____

RELAXATION

NUTRITION

CRAVINGS: _____

AVERSIONS: _____

NOTES: _____

DAILY WRAP-UP

MEDS / TESTS

tuesday

WEIGHT ☐ PRENATAL SUPPLEMENT ☐ KEGELS ☐☐

EXERCISE

CARDIO: _____

RPE / HR: _____

_____

STRENGTH: _____

_____

RELAXATION

NUTRITION

CRAVINGS: _____

AVERSIONS: _____

NOTES: _____

DAILY WRAP-UP

MEDS / TESTS

YOUR BABY THIS WEEK: Baby has hair follicles, budding fingernails, and even some of the swooshes and whorls that will one day be fingerprints. If baby is a girl, she also has ovaries by now; if baby's a boy, his testicles and scrotum are a done deal.

wednesday

WEIGHT ☐ PRENATAL SUPPLEMENT ☐ KEGELS ☐☐

EXERCISE

CARDIO: _____

RPE / HR: _____

_____

_____

STRENGTH: _____

_____

_____

RELAXATION

DAILY WRAP-UP

NUTRITION

CRAVINGS: _____

AVERSIONS: _____

NOTES: _____

MEDS / TESTS

_____

_____

_____

_____

thursday

WEIGHT ☐ PRENATAL SUPPLEMENT ☐ KEGELS ☐☐

EXERCISE

CARDIO: _____

RPE / HR: _____

_____

_____

STRENGTH: _____

_____

RELAXATION

DAILY WRAP-UP

NUTRITION

CRAVINGS: _____

AVERSIONS: _____

NOTES: _____

MEDS / TESTS

_____

_____

_____

_____

BY THE NUMBERS: 56,000: Number of extra calories it takes to create a baby. **150:** Number of extra calories per day mom needs to eat while pregnant in the first and second trimesters. **300:** Number of extra calories per day mom needs in the third trimester.

friday

WEIGHT [ ]   PRENATAL SUPPLEMENT [ ]   KEGELS [ ][ ]

EXERCISE

CARDIO:

RPE / HR:

STRENGTH:

RELAXATION

NUTRITION

CRAVINGS:

AVERSIONS:

NOTES:

DAILY WRAP-UP

MEDS / TESTS

saturday

WEIGHT [ ]   PRENATAL SUPPLEMENT [ ]   KEGELS [ ][ ]

EXERCISE

CARDIO:

RPE / HR:

STRENGTH:

RELAXATION

NUTRITION

CRAVINGS:

AVERSIONS:

NOTES:

DAILY WRAP-UP

MEDS / TESTS

> **"I'm not interested in being Wonder Woman in the delivery room. Give me drugs."**
> **— MADONNA**

sunday

WEIGHT [ ] PRENATAL SUPPLEMENT [ ] KEGELS [ ][ ]

EXERCISE

CARDIO: _____

RPE / HR: _____

_____

_____

STRENGTH: _____

_____

_____

RELAXATION

NUTRITION

CRAVINGS: _____

_____

AVERSIONS: _____

_____

NOTES: _____

_____

_____

DAILY WRAP-UP

MEDS / TESTS

_____

_____

_____

_____

weekly wrap-up

GOALS MET _____ EXCEEDED _____ MAYBE NEXT WEEK _____

EXERCISE TOTAL CARDIO SESSIONS [ ] TOTAL CARDIO HOURS [ ] TOTAL STRENGTH SESSIONS [ ]

NOTES _____

_____

_____

NUTRITION

REFLECTIONS ON THE WEEK

week
12

Dates: _____

Goals: _____

_____

_____

monday

WEIGHT		PRENATAL SUPPLEMENT		KEGELS		

EXERCISE

CARDIO: _____

RPE / HR: _____

_____

_____

STRENGTH: _____

_____

_____

RELAXATION

NUTRITION

CRAVINGS: _____

_____

AVERSIONS: _____

_____

NOTES: _____

_____

DAILY WRAP-UP

MEDS / TESTS

_____

_____

_____

_____

tuesday

WEIGHT		PRENATAL SUPPLEMENT		KEGELS		

EXERCISE

CARDIO: _____

RPE / HR: _____

_____

_____

STRENGTH: _____

_____

_____

RELAXATION

NUTRITION

CRAVINGS: _____

_____

AVERSIONS: _____

_____

NOTES: _____

_____

DAILY WRAP-UP

MEDS / TESTS

_____

_____

_____

_____

YOUR BABY THIS WEEK: A big week on the organ front: baby's thyroid, pancreas, and gall bladder have completed their development. Baby is now 3 inches long and more in proportion; whereas last month baby's head was half the size of her body, now her head is just one-third her size.

wednesday

WEIGHT ☐ PRENATAL SUPPLEMENT ☐ KEGELS ☐☐

EXERCISE

CARDIO:

RPE / HR:

STRENGTH:

RELAXATION

NUTRITION

CRAVINGS:

AVERSIONS:

NOTES:

DAILY WRAP-UP

MEDS / TESTS

thursday

WEIGHT ☐ PRENATAL SUPPLEMENT ☐ KEGELS ☐☐

EXERCISE

CARDIO:

RPE / HR:

STRENGTH:

RELAXATION

NUTRITION

CRAVINGS:

AVERSIONS:

NOTES:

DAILY WRAP-UP

MEDS / TESTS

DID YOU KNOW? Early in the pregnancy, the placenta produces amniotic fluid, which primarily serves as a cushion for junior. After about the fourth month of pregnancy, most amniotic fluid comes from the fetus peeing out and swallowing fluids in a tidy cycle.

friday

WEIGHT | PRENATAL SUPPLEMENT | KEGELS

EXERCISE

CARDIO:

RPE / HR:

STRENGTH:

RELAXATION

NUTRITION

CRAVINGS:

AVERSIONS:

NOTES:

DAILY WRAP-UP

MEDS / TESTS

saturday

WEIGHT | PRENATAL SUPPLEMENT | KEGELS

EXERCISE

CARDIO:

RPE / HR:

STRENGTH:

RELAXATION

NUTRITION

CRAVINGS:

AVERSIONS:

NOTES:

DAILY WRAP-UP

MEDS / TESTS

sunday

WEIGHT ☐ PRENATAL SUPPLEMENT ☐ KEGELS ☐☐

EXERCISE

CARDIO:

RPE / HR:

STRENGTH:

RELAXATION

NUTRITION

CRAVINGS:

AVERSIONS:

NOTES:

DAILY WRAP-UP

MEDS / TESTS

weekly wrap-up

GOALS   MET _____   EXCEEDED _____   MAYBE NEXT WEEK _____

EXERCISE   TOTAL CARDIO SESSIONS ☐   TOTAL CARDIO HOURS ☐   TOTAL STRENGTH SESSIONS ☐

NOTES _____

NUTRITION

REFLECTIONS ON THE WEEK

week 13

Dates:

Goals:

monday

WEIGHT ☐ PRENATAL SUPPLEMENT ☐ KEGELS ☐☐

EXERCISE

CARDIO:

RPE / HR:

STRENGTH:

RELAXATION

NUTRITION

CRAVINGS:

AVERSIONS:

NOTES:

DAILY WRAP-UP

MEDS / TESTS

tuesday

WEIGHT ☐ PRENATAL SUPPLEMENT ☐ KEGELS ☐☐

EXERCISE

CARDIO:

RPE / HR:

STRENGTH:

RELAXATION

NUTRITION

CRAVINGS:

AVERSIONS:

NOTES:

DAILY WRAP-UP

MEDS / TESTS

YOUR BABY THIS WEEK: Be sure to eat something yummy this week because baby's taste buds are now nearly as developed as yours. Baby will begin sampling the amniotic fluid, which carries tastes and smells from your diet.

wednesday

WEIGHT ☐ PRENATAL SUPPLEMENT ☐ KEGELS ☐☐

EXERCISE

CARDIO:

RPE / HR:

STRENGTH:

RELAXATION

NUTRITION

CRAVINGS:

AVERSIONS:

NOTES:

DAILY WRAP-UP

MEDS / TESTS

thursday

WEIGHT ☐ PRENATAL SUPPLEMENT ☐ KEGELS ☐☐

EXERCISE

CARDIO:

RPE / HR:

STRENGTH:

RELAXATION

NUTRITION

CRAVINGS:

AVERSIONS:

NOTES:

DAILY WRAP-UP

MEDS / TESTS

BY THE NUMBERS: **2.6:** Average birth rate in Utah, the nation's highest average. **1.7:** Average births per female resident of Maine, Massachusetts, and Vermont. **7.5:** Average number of children per woman in Niger, Africa — the highest fertility rate in the world. **1.3:** Birth rate in Italy and Spain.

friday

WEIGHT   PRENATAL SUPPLEMENT   KEGELS

EXERCISE

CARDIO:

RPE / HR:

STRENGTH:

RELAXATION

NUTRITION

CRAVINGS:

AVERSIONS:

NOTES:

DAILY WRAP-UP

MEDS / TESTS

saturday

WEIGHT   PRENATAL SUPPLEMENT   KEGELS

EXERCISE

CARDIO:

RPE / HR:

STRENGTH:

RELAXATION

NUTRITION

CRAVINGS:

AVERSIONS:

NOTES:

DAILY WRAP-UP

MEDS / TESTS

"Giving birth is like taking your lower lip and forcing it over your head."
— CAROL BURNETT

sunday

WEIGHT [ ] PRENATAL SUPPLEMENT [ ] KEGELS [ ][ ]

EXERCISE

CARDIO:

RPE / HR:

STRENGTH:

RELAXATION

NUTRITION

CRAVINGS:

AVERSIONS:

NOTES:

MEDS / TESTS

DAILY WRAP-UP

weekly wrap-up

GOALS   MET _____   EXCEEDED _____   MAYBE NEXT WEEK _____

EXERCISE   TOTAL CARDIO SESSIONS [ ]   TOTAL CARDIO HOURS [ ]   TOTAL STRENGTH SESSIONS [ ]

NOTES

NUTRITION

REFLECTIONS ON THE WEEK

week 14

Dates: _____

Goals: _____

monday

WEIGHT [ ] **PRENATAL SUPPLEMENT** [ ] **KEGELS** [ ][ ]

EXERCISE

CARDIO: _____

RPE / HR: _____

_____

_____

STRENGTH: _____

_____

_____

RELAXATION

NUTRITION

CRAVINGS: _____

AVERSIONS: _____

NOTES: _____

_____

DAILY WRAP-UP

MEDS / TESTS

_____

_____

_____

_____

tuesday

WEIGHT [ ] **PRENATAL SUPPLEMENT** [ ] **KEGELS** [ ][ ]

EXERCISE

CARDIO: _____

RPE / HR: _____

_____

_____

STRENGTH: _____

_____

_____

RELAXATION

NUTRITION

CRAVINGS: _____

AVERSIONS: _____

NOTES: _____

_____

DAILY WRAP-UP

MEDS / TESTS

_____

_____

_____

_____

YOUR BABY THIS WEEK: Baby is now about the size of a lime and has begun working out those tiny, gorgeous facial muscles by squinting, frowning, and grimacing. Eager to test-drive her growing arms and legs, baby is quite the mover and shaker now, though you won't feel the commotion just yet.

wednesday

WEIGHT ☐ PRENATAL SUPPLEMENT ☐ KEGELS ☐☐

EXERCISE

CARDIO:

RPE / HR:

STRENGTH:

RELAXATION

DAILY WRAP-UP

NUTRITION

CRAVINGS:

AVERSIONS:

NOTES:

MEDS / TESTS

thursday

WEIGHT ☐ PRENATAL SUPPLEMENT ☐ KEGELS ☐☐

EXERCISE

CARDIO:

RPE / HR:

STRENGTH:

RELAXATION

DAILY WRAP-UP

NUTRITION

CRAVINGS:

AVERSIONS:

NOTES:

MEDS / TESTS

DID YOU KNOW? Fetal thumb sucking can be seen via ultrasound as early as 12 weeks' gestation. By week 31 of gestation, a baby may have a callus on her thumb from sucking it.

friday

WEIGHT [ ] PRENATAL SUPPLEMENT [ ] KEGELS [|]

EXERCISE

CARDIO:

RPE / HR:

STRENGTH:

RELAXATION

NUTRITION

CRAVINGS:

AVERSIONS:

NOTES:

DAILY WRAP-UP

MEDS / TESTS

saturday

WEIGHT [ ] PRENATAL SUPPLEMENT [ ] KEGELS [|]

EXERCISE

CARDIO:

RPE / HR:

STRENGTH:

RELAXATION

NUTRITION

CRAVINGS:

AVERSIONS:

NOTES:

DAILY WRAP-UP

MEDS / TESTS

THROUGH THE AGES: In the 1500s, a Swiss farmer carried out the first recorded Cesarean delivery in which both the mother and baby survived. The first successful C-section using Western medical techniques took place around 1815 and is credited to a British female doctor who masqueraded as a man.

sunday

WEIGHT ☐ PRENATAL SUPPLEMENT ☐ KEGELS ☐☐

EXERCISE

CARDIO: _____

RPE / HR: _____

_____

_____

STRENGTH: _____

_____

_____

RELAXATION

NUTRITION

CRAVINGS: _____

AVERSIONS: _____

NOTES: _____

MEDS / TESTS

DAILY WRAP-UP

weekly wrap-up

GOALS   MET _____   EXCEEDED _____   MAYBE NEXT WEEK _____

EXERCISE   TOTAL CARDIO SESSIONS ☐   TOTAL CARDIO HOURS ☐   TOTAL STRENGTH SESSIONS ☐

NOTES _____

_____

_____

NUTRITION

REFLECTIONS ON THE WEEK

week
15

monday

WEIGHT   **PRENATAL SUPPLEMENT**   KEGELS

EXERCISE

CARDIO:

RPE / HR:

STRENGTH:

RELAXATION

NUTRITION

CRAVINGS:

AVERSIONS:

NOTES:

DAILY WRAP-UP

MEDS / TESTS

tuesday

WEIGHT   **PRENATAL SUPPLEMENT**   KEGELS

EXERCISE

CARDIO:

RPE / HR:

STRENGTH:

RELAXATION

NUTRITION

CRAVINGS:

AVERSIONS:

NOTES:

DAILY WRAP-UP

MEDS / TESTS

YOUR BABY THIS WEEK: Welcome to the second trimester! Baby's latest tricks: kicking, grasping, swallowing, toe curling, fist making, thumb wiggling. Though her eyelids are fused shut, baby can sense light now. To get her developing lungs in shape, baby is now inhaling and exhaling amniotic fluid.

wednesday

WEIGHT ☐ PRENATAL SUPPLEMENT ☐ KEGELS ☐☐

EXERCISE

CARDIO:

RPE / HR:

STRENGTH:

RELAXATION

NUTRITION

CRAVINGS:

AVERSIONS:

NOTES:

DAILY WRAP-UP

MEDS / TESTS

thursday

WEIGHT ☐ PRENATAL SUPPLEMENT ☐ KEGELS ☐☐

EXERCISE

CARDIO:

RPE / HR:

STRENGTH:

RELAXATION

NUTRITION

CRAVINGS:

AVERSIONS:

NOTES:

DAILY WRAP-UP

MEDS / TESTS

BY THE NUMBERS: 300: Number of bones that babies are born with. **206:** Number of bones a person has from age 12. You don't lose bones en route from childhood to adulthood. Some bones in the head and lower spine simply fuse together.

friday

WEIGHT [ ]   PRENATAL SUPPLEMENT [ ]   KEGELS [|]

EXERCISE _____

CARDIO: _____

RPE / HR: _____

_____

_____

STRENGTH: _____

_____

_____

RELAXATION

DAILY WRAP-UP

NUTRITION _____

CRAVINGS: _____

_____

AVERSIONS: _____

NOTES: _____

_____

MEDS / TESTS

_____

_____

_____

_____

saturday

WEIGHT [ ]   PRENATAL SUPPLEMENT [ ]   KEGELS [|]

EXERCISE _____

CARDIO: _____

RPE / HR: _____

_____

_____

STRENGTH: _____

_____

RELAXATION

DAILY WRAP-UP

NUTRITION _____

CRAVINGS: _____

_____

AVERSIONS: _____

NOTES: _____

_____

MEDS / TESTS

_____

_____

_____

_____

"If pregnancy were a book, they would cut the last two chapters."
— NORA EPHRON, in Heartburn

sunday

WEIGHT ☐   PRENATAL SUPPLEMENT ☐   KEGELS ☐ ☐

EXERCISE

CARDIO:

RPE / HR:

STRENGTH:

RELAXATION

NUTRITION

CRAVINGS:

AVERSIONS:

NOTES:

DAILY WRAP-UP

MEDS / TESTS

weekly wrap-up

GOALS   MET _____   EXCEEDED _____   MAYBE NEXT WEEK _____

EXERCISE   TOTAL CARDIO SESSIONS ☐   TOTAL CARDIO HOURS ☐   TOTAL STRENGTH SESSIONS ☐

NOTES

NUTRITION

REFLECTIONS ON THE WEEK

week 16

Dates:

Goals:

---

monday

WEIGHT ☐   PRENATAL SUPPLEMENT ☐   KEGELS ☐☐

EXERCISE

CARDIO:

RPE / HR:

STRENGTH:

RELAXATION

NUTRITION

CRAVINGS:

AVERSIONS:

NOTES:

DAILY WRAP-UP

MEDS / TESTS

---

tuesday

WEIGHT ☐   PRENATAL SUPPLEMENT ☐   KEGELS ☐☐

EXERCISE

CARDIO:

RPE / HR:

STRENGTH:

RELAXATION

NUTRITION

CRAVINGS:

AVERSIONS:

NOTES:

DAILY WRAP-UP

MEDS / TESTS

YOUR BABY THIS WEEK: Get ready for a future full of butterfly kisses: this week baby is making eyelashes! Baby is also experiencing a big growth spurt, weighing in around 5 ounces and measuring more than 4 inches long. All of baby's muscles and bones are in place.

wednesday

WEIGHT ☐ PRENATAL SUPPLEMENT ☐ KEGELS ☐☐

EXERCISE

CARDIO:

RPE / HR:

STRENGTH:

RELAXATION

NUTRITION

CRAVINGS:

AVERSIONS:

NOTES:

DAILY WRAP-UP

MEDS / TESTS

thursday

WEIGHT ☐ PRENATAL SUPPLEMENT ☐ KEGELS ☐☐

EXERCISE

CARDIO:

RPE / HR:

STRENGTH:

RELAXATION

NUTRITION

CRAVINGS:

AVERSIONS:

NOTES:

DAILY WRAP-UP

MEDS / TESTS

DID YOU KNOW? Human females are the only mammals that ovulate without realizing it and without any outward sign that the female is ready to conceive. We're also the only mammals whose breasts enlarge when pregnant.

friday

WEIGHT ☐   PRENATAL SUPPLEMENT ☐   KEGELS ☐ ☐

EXERCISE

CARDIO:

RPE / HR:

_____

_____

STRENGTH:

_____

_____

RELAXATION

NUTRITION

CRAVINGS:

_____

AVERSIONS:

_____

NOTES:

_____

DAILY WRAP-UP

MEDS / TESTS

saturday

WEIGHT ☐   PRENATAL SUPPLEMENT ☐   KEGELS ☐ ☐

EXERCISE

CARDIO:

RPE / HR:

_____

_____

STRENGTH:

_____

_____

RELAXATION

NUTRITION

CRAVINGS:

_____

AVERSIONS:

_____

NOTES:

_____

DAILY WRAP-UP

MEDS / TESTS

THROUGH THE AGES: John was the number 1 popular boy's name in the 1880s and number 3 in the 1960s. By the 1990s, John had dropped to number 14. Mary, the most popular girl's name in the 1880s, was number 2 in the 1960s but by the 1990s had dropped out of the top 20.

sunday

WEIGHT ☐ PRENATAL SUPPLEMENT ☐ KEGELS ☐ ☐

EXERCISE

CARDIO:

RPE / HR:

STRENGTH:

RELAXATION

NUTRITION

CRAVINGS:

AVERSIONS:

NOTES:

DAILY WRAP-UP

MEDS / TESTS

weekly wrap-up

GOALS MET _____ EXCEEDED _____ MAYBE NEXT WEEK _____

EXERCISE TOTAL CARDIO SESSIONS ☐ TOTAL CARDIO HOURS ☐ TOTAL STRENGTH SESSIONS ☐

NOTES

NUTRITION

REFLECTIONS ON THE WEEK

week
17

Dates: _____

Goals: _____
_____
_____

monday

WEIGHT [ ]   PRENATAL SUPPLEMENT [ ]   KEGELS [ ][ ]

EXERCISE

CARDIO: _____

RPE / HR: _____

_____

_____

STRENGTH: _____

_____

_____

RELAXATION

NUTRITION

CRAVINGS: _____

_____

AVERSIONS: _____

_____

NOTES: _____

_____

DAILY WRAP-UP

MEDS / TESTS

_____

_____

_____

_____

tuesday

WEIGHT [ ]   PRENATAL SUPPLEMENT [ ]   KEGELS [ ][ ]

EXERCISE

CARDIO: _____

RPE / HR: _____

_____

_____

STRENGTH: _____

_____

_____

RELAXATION

NUTRITION

CRAVINGS: _____

_____

AVERSIONS: _____

_____

NOTES: _____

_____

DAILY WRAP-UP

MEDS / TESTS

_____

_____

_____

_____

YOUR BABY THIS WEEK: Baby really cutens up this week as her eyes move forward, and she sprouts ears. Lanugo, fine hair that grows to protect the skin, now appears on her head and body. Baby is now approximately the same size as the placenta but will soon grow larger.

wednesday

WEIGHT ☐ PRENATAL SUPPLEMENT ☐ KEGELS ☐☐

EXERCISE

CARDIO:

RPE / HR:

STRENGTH:

RELAXATION

NUTRITION

CRAVINGS:

AVERSIONS:

NOTES:

DAILY WRAP-UP

MEDS / TESTS

thursday

WEIGHT ☐ PRENATAL SUPPLEMENT ☐ KEGELS ☐☐

EXERCISE

CARDIO:

RPE / HR:

STRENGTH:

RELAXATION

NUTRITION

CRAVINGS:

AVERSIONS:

NOTES:

DAILY WRAP-UP

MEDS / TESTS

BY THE NUMBERS: 74: Percent increase in twin births from 1980 to 2000, due to increase in fertility treatments and delayed age of birth mothers. **3:** Percent of all babies who were born as a twin or higher-order multiple in 2000. **1.2:** Historical rate of twin pregnancies.

friday

WEIGHT ☐   PRENATAL SUPPLEMENT ☐   KEGELS ☐☐

EXERCISE

CARDIO:

RPE / HR:

STRENGTH:

RELAXATION

NUTRITION

CRAVINGS:

AVERSIONS:

NOTES:

DAILY WRAP-UP

MEDS / TESTS

saturday

WEIGHT ☐   PRENATAL SUPPLEMENT ☐   KEGELS ☐☐

EXERCISE

CARDIO:

RPE / HR:

STRENGTH:

RELAXATION

NUTRITION

CRAVINGS:

AVERSIONS:

NOTES:

DAILY WRAP-UP

MEDS / TESTS

"A ship under sail and a big-bellied woman,
  Are the handsomest two things that can be seen common."

— BENJAMIN FRANKLIN

sunday

WEIGHT ☐   PRENATAL SUPPLEMENT ☐   KEGELS ☐☐

EXERCISE

CARDIO:

RPE / HR:

STRENGTH:

RELAXATION

NUTRITION

CRAVINGS:

AVERSIONS:

NOTES:

DAILY WRAP-UP

MEDS / TESTS

weekly wrap-up

GOALS   MET _____   EXCEEDED _____   MAYBE NEXT WEEK _____

EXERCISE   TOTAL CARDIO SESSIONS ☐   TOTAL CARDIO HOURS ☐   TOTAL STRENGTH SESSIONS ☐

NOTES

NUTRITION

REFLECTIONS ON THE WEEK

week 18

Dates: _____

Goals: _____

_____

_____

monday

WEIGHT [ ]   **PRENATAL SUPPLEMENT** [ ]   KEGELS [|]

EXERCISE

CARDIO: _____

RPE / HR: _____

_____

_____

STRENGTH: _____

_____

_____

RELAXATION

DAILY WRAP-UP

NUTRITION

CRAVINGS: _____

AVERSIONS: _____

NOTES: _____

_____

MEDS / TESTS

_____

_____

_____

_____

tuesday

WEIGHT [ ]   **PRENATAL SUPPLEMENT** [ ]   KEGELS [|]

EXERCISE

CARDIO: _____

RPE / HR: _____

_____

_____

STRENGTH: _____

_____

_____

RELAXATION

DAILY WRAP-UP

NUTRITION

CRAVINGS: _____

AVERSIONS: _____

NOTES: _____

_____

MEDS / TESTS

_____

_____

_____

_____

YOUR BABY THIS WEEK: Hello in there! This week your baby's hearing is fully functional. The soundtrack of her life includes your heartbeat and blood pumping through the umbilical cord, plus muffled noises from the outside world. Baby now has **200** of the **300** bones she will have at birth; many of these have begun to harden and are visible via ultrasound.

wednesday

WEIGHT [ ]   **PRENATAL SUPPLEMENT** [ ]   KEGELS [ ][ ]

EXERCISE

CARDIO:

RPE / HR:

_____

_____

STRENGTH:

_____

RELAXATION

DAILY WRAP-UP

NUTRITION

CRAVINGS:

_____

AVERSIONS:

_____

NOTES:

_____

MEDS / TESTS

_____

_____

_____

_____

thursday

WEIGHT [ ]   **PRENATAL SUPPLEMENT** [ ]   KEGELS [ ][ ]

EXERCISE

CARDIO:

RPE / HR:

_____

_____

STRENGTH:

_____

RELAXATION

DAILY WRAP-UP

NUTRITION

CRAVINGS:

_____

AVERSIONS:

_____

NOTES:

_____

MEDS / TESTS

_____

_____

_____

_____

DID YOU KNOW? Caucasian babies are always born with blue eyes. The color can change from within a few moments of delivery up to two years after birth. All babies are colorblind at birth.

friday

WEIGHT [ ]   PRENATAL SUPPLEMENT [ ]   KEGELS [|]

EXERCISE

CARDIO:

RPE / HR:

STRENGTH:

RELAXATION

DAILY WRAP-UP

NUTRITION

CRAVINGS:

AVERSIONS:

NOTES:

MEDS / TESTS

saturday

WEIGHT [ ]   PRENATAL SUPPLEMENT [ ]   KEGELS [|]

EXERCISE

CARDIO:

RPE / HR:

STRENGTH:

RELAXATION

DAILY WRAP-UP

NUTRITION

CRAVINGS:

AVERSIONS:

NOTES:

MEDS / TESTS

THROUGH THE AGES: In middle-class circles in nineteenth-century Britain, pregnancy was too delicate a subject to be discussed in mixed company. Pregnant women concealed their increasing size with voluminous clothes, shawls, scarves, and corsetry.

sunday

WEIGHT [ ] PRENATAL SUPPLEMENT [ ] KEGELS [ ][ ]

EXERCISE

CARDIO:

RPE / HR:

_____

_____

STRENGTH:

_____

_____

RELAXATION

NUTRITION

CRAVINGS:

_____

AVERSIONS:

_____

NOTES:

_____

_____

_____

DAILY WRAP-UP

MEDS / TESTS

_____

_____

_____

_____

weekly wrap-up

GOALS   MET _____   EXCEEDED _____   MAYBE NEXT WEEK _____

EXERCISE   TOTAL CARDIO SESSIONS [ ]   TOTAL CARDIO HOURS [ ]   TOTAL STRENGTH SESSIONS [ ]

NOTES _____

_____

_____

NUTRITION

REFLECTIONS ON THE WEEK

week 19

Dates: _____

Goals: _____

_____

_____

monday

WEIGHT [ ]   **PRENATAL SUPPLEMENT** [ ]   KEGELS [ ][ ]

EXERCISE

CARDIO: _____

RPE / HR: _____

_____

_____

STRENGTH: _____

_____

_____

RELAXATION

DAILY WRAP-UP

NUTRITION

CRAVINGS: _____

_____

AVERSIONS: _____

_____

NOTES: _____

_____

MEDS / TESTS

_____

_____

_____

_____

tuesday

WEIGHT [ ]   **PRENATAL SUPPLEMENT** [ ]   KEGELS [ ][ ]

EXERCISE

CARDIO: _____

RPE / HR: _____

_____

_____

STRENGTH: _____

_____

_____

RELAXATION

DAILY WRAP-UP

NUTRITION

CRAVINGS: _____

_____

AVERSIONS: _____

_____

NOTES: _____

_____

MEDS / TESTS

_____

_____

_____

_____

YOUR BABY THIS WEEK: Baby is now the size of a cucumber, with a body that's almost completely proportionate. You may begin to feel small fetal movements and flutters known as "quickening." If baby is a girl, miniature follicles are busy developing in her ovaries.

wednesday

WEIGHT ☐ PRENATAL SUPPLEMENT ☐ KEGELS ☐☐

EXERCISE

CARDIO:

RPE / HR:

_____

_____

STRENGTH:

_____

RELAXATION

NUTRITION

CRAVINGS:

_____

AVERSIONS:

_____

NOTES:

_____

_____

DAILY WRAP-UP

MEDS / TESTS

_____

_____

_____

_____

thursday

WEIGHT ☐ PRENATAL SUPPLEMENT ☐ KEGELS ☐☐

EXERCISE

CARDIO:

RPE / HR:

_____

_____

STRENGTH:

_____

RELAXATION

NUTRITION

CRAVINGS:

_____

AVERSIONS:

_____

NOTES:

_____

_____

DAILY WRAP-UP

MEDS / TESTS

_____

_____

_____

_____

friday

WEIGHT ☐ PRENATAL SUPPLEMENT ☐ KEGELS ☐☐

EXERCISE

CARDIO:

RPE / HR:

STRENGTH:

RELAXATION

DAILY WRAP-UP

NUTRITION

CRAVINGS:

AVERSIONS:

NOTES:

MEDS / TESTS

saturday

WEIGHT ☐ PRENATAL SUPPLEMENT ☐ KEGELS ☐☐

EXERCISE

CARDIO:

RPE / HR:

STRENGTH:

RELAXATION

DAILY WRAP-UP

NUTRITION

CRAVINGS:

AVERSIONS:

NOTES:

MEDS / TESTS

"Life is tough enough without having someone kick you from the inside."

— RITA RUDNER

sunday

WEIGHT ☐ PRENATAL SUPPLEMENT ☐ KEGELS ☐ ☐

EXERCISE

CARDIO: _____

RPE / HR: _____

_____

_____

STRENGTH: _____

_____

_____

RELAXATION

NUTRITION

CRAVINGS: _____

AVERSIONS: _____

NOTES: _____

_____

DAILY WRAP-UP

MEDS / TESTS

_____

_____

_____

_____

weekly wrap-up

GOALS MET _____ EXCEEDED _____ MAYBE NEXT WEEK _____

EXERCISE TOTAL CARDIO SESSIONS ☐ TOTAL CARDIO HOURS ☐ TOTAL STRENGTH SESSIONS ☐

NOTES _____

_____

_____

NUTRITION

REFLECTIONS ON THE WEEK

week
20

Dates: _____

Goals: _____
_____
_____

monday

WEIGHT [ ] **PRENATAL SUPPLEMENT** [ ] KEGELS [ ][ ]

EXERCISE

CARDIO: _____

RPE / HR: _____
_____
_____

STRENGTH: _____
_____
_____

RELAXATION

DAILY WRAP-UP

NUTRITION

CRAVINGS: _____
_____

AVERSIONS: _____
_____

NOTES: _____
_____

MEDS / TESTS
_____
_____
_____
_____

tuesday

WEIGHT [ ] **PRENATAL SUPPLEMENT** [ ] KEGELS [ ][ ]

EXERCISE

CARDIO: _____

RPE / HR: _____
_____
_____

STRENGTH: _____
_____

RELAXATION

DAILY WRAP-UP

NUTRITION

CRAVINGS: _____
_____

AVERSIONS: _____
_____

NOTES: _____
_____

MEDS / TESTS
_____
_____
_____
_____

YOUR BABY THIS WEEK: At this point, baby is about 10 inches long and tips the scales at about 10 ounces. She's producing vernix, a creamy white substance designed to protect her delicate skin from the harsh amniotic fluid. New moms used to use it as a hand lotion because of its smooth quality.

wednesday

WEIGHT ☐ PRENATAL SUPPLEMENT ☐ KEGELS ☐☐

EXERCISE

CARDIO:

RPE / HR:

STRENGTH:

RELAXATION

NUTRITION

CRAVINGS:

AVERSIONS:

NOTES:

DAILY WRAP-UP

MEDS / TESTS

thursday

WEIGHT ☐ PRENATAL SUPPLEMENT ☐ KEGELS ☐☐

EXERCISE

CARDIO:

RPE / HR:

STRENGTH:

RELAXATION

NUTRITION

CRAVINGS:

AVERSIONS:

NOTES:

DAILY WRAP-UP

MEDS / TESTS

DID YOU KNOW? One in every 2,000 babies is born with a tooth. This extra tooth will fall out when the baby tooth erupts, but sometimes may need to be removed, to avoid the risk of choking if it's loose. A baby's first tooth typically doesn't appear until 3 to 10 months after birth.

friday

WEIGHT ☐   PRENATAL SUPPLEMENT ☐   KEGELS ☐☐

EXERCISE

CARDIO:

RPE / HR:

STRENGTH:

RELAXATION

NUTRITION

CRAVINGS:

AVERSIONS:

NOTES:

DAILY WRAP-UP

MEDS / TESTS

saturday

WEIGHT ☐   PRENATAL SUPPLEMENT ☐   KEGELS ☐☐

EXERCISE

CARDIO:

RPE / HR:

STRENGTH:

RELAXATION

NUTRITION

CRAVINGS:

AVERSIONS:

NOTES:

DAILY WRAP-UP

MEDS / TESTS

THROUGH THE AGES: In colonial America, it was common for the laboring woman to be seated on her husband's lap while he was seated on a chair. Labor pain was thought to be relieved by opening the windows or setting the horses free from the stable.

sunday

WEIGHT ☐   PRENATAL SUPPLEMENT ☐   KEGELS ☐ ☐

EXERCISE

CARDIO:

RPE / HR:

STRENGTH:

RELAXATION

NUTRITION

CRAVINGS:

AVERSIONS:

NOTES:

MEDS / TESTS

DAILY WRAP-UP

weekly wrap-up

GOALS   MET _____   EXCEEDED _____   MAYBE NEXT WEEK _____

EXERCISE   TOTAL CARDIO SESSIONS ☐   TOTAL CARDIO HOURS ☐   TOTAL STRENGTH SESSIONS ☐

NOTES

NUTRITION

REFLECTIONS ON THE WEEK

week 21

Dates: _____

Goals: _____
_____
_____

monday

WEIGHT [ ]   PRENATAL SUPPLEMENT [ ]   KEGELS [ ][ ]

EXERCISE

CARDIO: _____

RPE / HR: _____

_____

_____

STRENGTH: _____

_____

RELAXATION

DAILY WRAP-UP

NUTRITION

CRAVINGS: _____

_____

AVERSIONS: _____

_____

NOTES: _____

_____

MEDS / TESTS

_____

_____

_____

_____

tuesday

WEIGHT [ ]   PRENATAL SUPPLEMENT [ ]   KEGELS [ ][ ]

EXERCISE

CARDIO: _____

RPE / HR: _____

_____

_____

STRENGTH: _____

_____

RELAXATION

DAILY WRAP-UP

NUTRITION

CRAVINGS: _____

_____

AVERSIONS: _____

_____

NOTES: _____

_____

MEDS / TESTS

_____

_____

_____

_____

YOUR BABY THIS WEEK: Congratulations! Your baby is officially halfway baked! Until now your baby's liver and spleen have been manufacturing all of the blood cells, but now her bone marrow has taken on the major part of that job. Meanwhile, baby's heartbeat can be detected via a stethoscope.

wednesday

WEIGHT ☐ PRENATAL SUPPLEMENT ☐ KEGELS ☐ ☐

EXERCISE

CARDIO:

RPE / HR:

STRENGTH:

RELAXATION

NUTRITION

CRAVINGS:

AVERSIONS:

NOTES:

DAILY WRAP-UP

MEDS / TESTS

thursday

WEIGHT ☐ PRENATAL SUPPLEMENT ☐ KEGELS ☐ ☐

EXERCISE

CARDIO:

RPE / HR:

STRENGTH:

RELAXATION

NUTRITION

CRAVINGS:

AVERSIONS:

NOTES:

DAILY WRAP-UP

MEDS / TESTS

BY THE NUMBERS: 6: Percent of U.S. babies delivered by midwives in 1975. **8:** Percent delivered by midwives in 2003. **80:** Percent of newborns delivered by midwives worldwide. **98:** Percent of people alive today who were born at home, worldwide.

friday

WEIGHT ☐ PRENATAL SUPPLEMENT ☐ KEGELS ☐☐

EXERCISE

CARDIO:

RPE / HR:

STRENGTH:

RELAXATION

NUTRITION

CRAVINGS:

AVERSIONS:

NOTES:

DAILY WRAP-UP

MEDS / TESTS

saturday

WEIGHT ☐ PRENATAL SUPPLEMENT ☐ KEGELS ☐☐

EXERCISE

CARDIO:

RPE / HR:

STRENGTH:

RELAXATION

NUTRITION

CRAVINGS:

AVERSIONS:

NOTES:

DAILY WRAP-UP

MEDS / TESTS

"So I went over to my wife and . . . said, "I love you, very very much, dear. You just . . . had . . . a lizard. I mean, because the thing changed colors, like, five times!" — **BILL COSBY**, in the hospital at the birth of his first child

sunday

WEIGHT ☐ PRENATAL SUPPLEMENT ☐ KEGELS ☐☐

EXERCISE

CARDIO: _____

RPE / HR: _____

_____

_____

STRENGTH: _____

_____

RELAXATION

NUTRITION

CRAVINGS: _____

_____

AVERSIONS: _____

_____

NOTES: _____

_____

_____

DAILY WRAP-UP

MEDS / TESTS

_____

_____

_____

_____

weekly wrap-up

GOALS   MET _____   EXCEEDED _____   MAYBE NEXT WEEK _____

EXERCISE   TOTAL CARDIO SESSIONS ☐   TOTAL CARDIO HOURS ☐   TOTAL STRENGTH SESSIONS ☐

NOTES _____

_____

_____

NUTRITION

REFLECTIONS ON THE WEEK

week 22

Dates: _____

Goals: _____
_____
_____

monday

WEIGHT [ ]   PRENATAL SUPPLEMENT [ ]   KEGELS [ ][ ]

EXERCISE

CARDIO: _____

RPE / HR: _____

_____

STRENGTH: _____

_____

RELAXATION

DAILY WRAP-UP

NUTRITION

CRAVINGS: _____

AVERSIONS: _____

NOTES: _____

MEDS / TESTS

_____
_____
_____
_____

tuesday

WEIGHT [ ]   PRENATAL SUPPLEMENT [ ]   KEGELS [ ][ ]

EXERCISE

CARDIO: _____

RPE / HR: _____

_____

STRENGTH: _____

_____

RELAXATION

DAILY WRAP-UP

NUTRITION

CRAVINGS: _____

AVERSIONS: _____

NOTES: _____

MEDS / TESTS

_____
_____
_____
_____

YOUR BABY THIS WEEK: Did you have Indian food for dinner, or maybe Thai? Baby will know it; her taste buds are developed enough to distinguish different flavors. Baby also can hear more clearly because her inner-ear bones are mature enough to detect vibrations.

wednesday

WEIGHT ☐   PRENATAL SUPPLEMENT ☐   KEGELS ☐☐

EXERCISE

CARDIO:

RPE / HR:

STRENGTH:

RELAXATION

DAILY WRAP-UP

NUTRITION

CRAVINGS:

AVERSIONS:

NOTES:

MEDS / TESTS

thursday

WEIGHT ☐   PRENATAL SUPPLEMENT ☐   KEGELS ☐☐

EXERCISE

CARDIO:

RPE / HR:

STRENGTH:

RELAXATION

DAILY WRAP-UP

NUTRITION

CRAVINGS:

AVERSIONS:

NOTES:

MEDS / TESTS

DID YOU KNOW? In utero, babies' ears are so sensitive to external sounds that they even recognize the language spoken around them. After birth, babies suck more vigorously if they hear recordings of people speaking in their native tongue than they do if they hear foreign speakers.

friday

WEIGHT ☐ PRENATAL SUPPLEMENT ☐ KEGELS ☐☐

EXERCISE

CARDIO:

RPE / HR:

STRENGTH:

RELAXATION

NUTRITION

CRAVINGS:

AVERSIONS:

NOTES:

DAILY WRAP-UP

MEDS / TESTS

saturday

WEIGHT ☐ PRENATAL SUPPLEMENT ☐ KEGELS ☐☐

EXERCISE

CARDIO:

RPE / HR:

STRENGTH:

RELAXATION

NUTRITION

CRAVINGS:

AVERSIONS:

NOTES:

DAILY WRAP-UP

MEDS / TESTS

THROUGH THE AGES: It wasn't until 1974 that the American College of Obstetricians and Gynecologists endorsed the presence of fathers at childbirth. Ninety-five percent of men now attend the birth of their child, compared to only 65 percent in 1965.

sunday

WEIGHT ☐ PRENATAL SUPPLEMENT ☐ KEGELS ☐☐

EXERCISE

CARDIO:

RPE / HR:

STRENGTH:

RELAXATION

NUTRITION

CRAVINGS:

AVERSIONS:

NOTES:

MEDS / TESTS

DAILY WRAP-UP

weekly wrap-up

GOALS   MET _____   EXCEEDED _____   MAYBE NEXT WEEK _____

EXERCISE   TOTAL CARDIO SESSIONS ☐   TOTAL CARDIO HOURS ☐   TOTAL STRENGTH SESSIONS ☐

NOTES

NUTRITION

REFLECTIONS ON THE WEEK

week 23

Dates:

Goals:

monday

WEIGHT ☐ PRENATAL SUPPLEMENT ☐ KEGELS ☐☐

EXERCISE

CARDIO:

RPE / HR:

STRENGTH:

RELAXATION

DAILY WRAP-UP

NUTRITION

CRAVINGS:

AVERSIONS:

NOTES:

MEDS / TESTS

tuesday

WEIGHT ☐ PRENATAL SUPPLEMENT ☐ KEGELS ☐☐

EXERCISE

CARDIO:

RPE / HR:

STRENGTH:

RELAXATION

DAILY WRAP-UP

NUTRITION

CRAVINGS:

AVERSIONS:

NOTES:

MEDS / TESTS

YOUR BABY THIS WEEK: You may really begin to understand the phrase "Sock it to me, baby" this week since your baby now has the ability to make a fist and might decide to give your uterine wall a good punch! Baby is about 11 inches long and weighs just more than 1 pound.

wednesday

WEIGHT ☐ PRENATAL SUPPLEMENT ☐ KEGELS ☐☐

EXERCISE _____

CARDIO: _____

RPE / HR: _____

_____

_____

STRENGTH: _____

_____

_____

RELAXATION

DAILY WRAP-UP

NUTRITION _____

CRAVINGS: _____

_____

AVERSIONS: _____

_____

NOTES: _____

_____

MEDS / TESTS

_____

_____

_____

_____

thursday

WEIGHT ☐ PRENATAL SUPPLEMENT ☐ KEGELS ☐☐

EXERCISE _____

CARDIO: _____

RPE / HR: _____

_____

_____

STRENGTH: _____

_____

_____

RELAXATION

DAILY WRAP-UP

NUTRITION _____

CRAVINGS: _____

_____

AVERSIONS: _____

_____

NOTES: _____

_____

MEDS / TESTS

_____

_____

_____

_____

BY THE NUMBERS: 48: Percent of Brazilian babies delivered via Cesarean. **26:** Percent of U.S. babies delivered by Cesarean. **15 to 17:** Cesarean birth rates in Scandivania. **10 to 15:** Percent of births in which C-sections are medically necessary, according to the World Health Organization.

friday

WEIGHT ☐ PRENATAL SUPPLEMENT ☐ KEGELS ☐ ☐

EXERCISE

CARDIO:

RPE / HR:

STRENGTH:

RELAXATION

DAILY WRAP-UP

NUTRITION

CRAVINGS:

AVERSIONS:

NOTES:

MEDS / TESTS

saturday

WEIGHT ☐ PRENATAL SUPPLEMENT ☐ KEGELS ☐ ☐

EXERCISE

CARDIO:

RPE / HR:

STRENGTH:

RELAXATION

DAILY WRAP-UP

NUTRITION

CRAVINGS:

AVERSIONS:

NOTES:

MEDS / TESTS

> "I already know how to breathe, and I'm the last person that needs to learn how to push."
> — CANDICE BERGEN, as Murphy Brown, in labor

sunday

WEIGHT ☐ PRENATAL SUPPLEMENT ☐ KEGELS ☐☐

EXERCISE

CARDIO:

RPE / HR:

STRENGTH:

RELAXATION

NUTRITION

CRAVINGS:

AVERSIONS:

NOTES:

DAILY WRAP-UP

MEDS / TESTS

weekly wrap-up

GOALS   MET _____   EXCEEDED _____   MAYBE NEXT WEEK _____

EXERCISE   TOTAL CARDIO SESSIONS ☐   TOTAL CARDIO HOURS ☐   TOTAL STRENGTH SESSIONS ☐

NOTES _____

_____

_____

NUTRITION

REFLECTIONS ON THE WEEK

week
24

Dates: _____

Goals: _____
_____
_____

monday

WEIGHT [ ] **PRENATAL SUPPLEMENT** [ ] **KEGELS** [ ][ ]

EXERCISE

CARDIO: _____

RPE / HR: _____

_____

_____

STRENGTH: _____

_____

_____

RELAXATION

DAILY WRAP-UP

NUTRITION

CRAVINGS: _____

_____

AVERSIONS: _____

_____

NOTES: _____

_____

MEDS / TESTS

_____

_____

_____

_____

_____

tuesday

WEIGHT [ ] **PRENATAL SUPPLEMENT** [ ] **KEGELS** [ ][ ]

EXERCISE

CARDIO: _____

RPE / HR: _____

_____

_____

STRENGTH: _____

_____

_____

RELAXATION

DAILY WRAP-UP

NUTRITION

CRAVINGS: _____

_____

AVERSIONS: _____

_____

NOTES: _____

_____

MEDS / TESTS

_____

_____

_____

_____

_____

YOUR BABY THIS WEEK: Your baby is almost completely formed and would have a better than 50 percent chance of surviving with intensive care if you gave birth prematurely. Her skin is thin, translucent, and wrinkled, and her brain is growing rapidly. She loves to yank on her umbilical cord.

wednesday

WEIGHT [ ] PRENATAL SUPPLEMENT [ ] KEGELS [|]

EXERCISE _____

CARDIO: _____

RPE / HR: _____

_____

_____

STRENGTH: _____

_____

_____

RELAXATION

NUTRITION _____

CRAVINGS: _____

_____

AVERSIONS: _____

_____

NOTES: _____

DAILY WRAP-UP

MEDS / TESTS _____

_____

_____

_____

_____

thursday

WEIGHT [ ] PRENATAL SUPPLEMENT [ ] KEGELS [|]

EXERCISE _____

CARDIO: _____

RPE / HR: _____

_____

_____

STRENGTH: _____

_____

_____

RELAXATION

NUTRITION _____

CRAVINGS: _____

_____

AVERSIONS: _____

_____

NOTES: _____

DAILY WRAP-UP

MEDS / TESTS _____

_____

_____

_____

_____

DID YOU KNOW? All those kicks and somersaults aren't just to keep you awake at night. They play a key role in the development of your baby's joint shape and structure and in defining the limbs' range of motion.

friday

WEIGHT ☐   PRENATAL SUPPLEMENT ☐   KEGELS ☐☐

EXERCISE

CARDIO:

RPE / HR:

STRENGTH:

RELAXATION

NUTRITION

CRAVINGS:

AVERSIONS:

NOTES:

MEDS / TESTS

DAILY WRAP-UP

saturday

WEIGHT ☐   PRENATAL SUPPLEMENT ☐   KEGELS ☐☐

EXERCISE

CARDIO:

RPE / HR:

STRENGTH:

RELAXATION

NUTRITION

CRAVINGS:

AVERSIONS:

NOTES:

MEDS / TESTS

DAILY WRAP-UP

THROUGH THE AGES: To speed up labor in the Middle Ages, everyone in the household would open cupboards and drawers, unlock chests, and untie knots — all symbolic of opening the womb. In Europe in the late nineteenth century, ringing of church bells was thought to hasten delivery.

sunday

WEIGHT ☐   PRENATAL SUPPLEMENT ☐   KEGELS ☐☐

EXERCISE

CARDIO:

RPE / HR:

STRENGTH:

RELAXATION

NUTRITION

CRAVINGS:

AVERSIONS:

NOTES:

MEDS / TESTS

DAILY WRAP-UP

weekly wrap-up

GOALS   MET _____   EXCEEDED _____   MAYBE NEXT WEEK _____

EXERCISE   TOTAL CARDIO SESSIONS ☐   TOTAL CARDIO HOURS ☐   TOTAL STRENGTH SESSIONS ☐

NOTES

NUTRITION

REFLECTIONS ON THE WEEK

week
25

Dates: _____

Goals: _____
_____
_____

monday

WEIGHT [ ] **PRENATAL SUPPLEMENT** [ ] **KEGELS** [|]

EXERCISE

CARDIO: _____

RPE / HR: _____

_____

STRENGTH: _____

_____

RELAXATION

DAILY WRAP-UP

NUTRITION

CRAVINGS: _____

AVERSIONS: _____

NOTES: _____

_____

MEDS / TESTS

_____
_____
_____
_____

tuesday

WEIGHT [ ] **PRENATAL SUPPLEMENT** [ ] **KEGELS** [|]

EXERCISE

CARDIO: _____

RPE / HR: _____

_____

STRENGTH: _____

_____

RELAXATION

DAILY WRAP-UP

NUTRITION

CRAVINGS: _____

AVERSIONS: _____

NOTES: _____

_____

MEDS / TESTS

_____
_____
_____
_____

YOUR BABY THIS WEEK: If your belly begins to jump, no worries. Your little one probably has the hiccups, which is really nothing more than a reflex in fetuses. Your babe now weighs about 1½ pounds and is beginning to pack on some baby fat. Her fingernails and toenails are lengthening.

wednesday

WEIGHT ☐ PRENATAL SUPPLEMENT ☐ KEGELS ☐☐

EXERCISE

CARDIO:

RPE / HR:

STRENGTH:

RELAXATION

NUTRITION

CRAVINGS:

AVERSIONS:

NOTES:

MEDS / TESTS

DAILY WRAP-UP

thursday

WEIGHT ☐ PRENATAL SUPPLEMENT ☐ KEGELS ☐☐

EXERCISE

CARDIO:

RPE / HR:

STRENGTH:

RELAXATION

NUTRITION

CRAVINGS:

AVERSIONS:

NOTES:

MEDS / TESTS

DAILY WRAP-UP

BY THE NUMBERS: 4: The average number of births per woman in the United States in 1900. **2.2:** The fertility rate during the Great Depression. **3.7:** The postwar fertility rate, peaking in 1957. **2.0:** Average births per woman over the last 20 years.

friday

WEIGHT

PRENATAL SUPPLEMENT

KEGELS

EXERCISE

CARDIO:

RPE / HR:

STRENGTH:

RELAXATION

NUTRITION

CRAVINGS:

AVERSIONS:

NOTES:

DAILY WRAP-UP

MEDS / TESTS

saturday

WEIGHT

PRENATAL SUPPLEMENT

KEGELS

EXERCISE

CARDIO:

RPE / HR:

STRENGTH:

RELAXATION

NUTRITION

CRAVINGS:

AVERSIONS:

NOTES:

DAILY WRAP-UP

MEDS / TESTS

"A child is a curly, dimpled lunatic." — RALPH WALDO EMERSON

sunday

WEIGHT [ ]   PRENATAL SUPPLEMENT [ ]   KEGELS [ ][ ]

EXERCISE

CARDIO:

RPE / HR:

STRENGTH:

RELAXATION

NUTRITION

CRAVINGS:

AVERSIONS:

NOTES:

DAILY WRAP-UP

MEDS / TESTS

weekly wrap-up

GOALS   MET _____   EXCEEDED _____   MAYBE NEXT WEEK _____

EXERCISE   TOTAL CARDIO SESSIONS [ ]   TOTAL CARDIO HOURS [ ]   TOTAL STRENGTH SESSIONS [ ]

NOTES

NUTRITION

REFLECTIONS ON THE WEEK

week 26

Dates:

Goals:

monday

WEIGHT ☐ PRENATAL SUPPLEMENT ☐ KEGELS ☐☐

EXERCISE

CARDIO:

RPE / HR:

STRENGTH:

RELAXATION

DAILY WRAP-UP

NUTRITION

CRAVINGS:

AVERSIONS:

NOTES:

MEDS / TESTS

tuesday

WEIGHT ☐ PRENATAL SUPPLEMENT ☐ KEGELS ☐☐

EXERCISE

CARDIO:

RPE / HR:

STRENGTH:

RELAXATION

DAILY WRAP-UP

NUTRITION

CRAVINGS:

AVERSIONS:

NOTES:

MEDS / TESTS

YOUR BABY THIS WEEK: Those beautiful peepers will pop open by the end of the week and probably even blink a time or two. At birth, vision will be perfectly focused from 8 to 12 inches. Baby weighs almost 2 pounds.

wednesday

WEIGHT ☐ PRENATAL SUPPLEMENT ☐ KEGELS ☐☐

EXERCISE

CARDIO:

RPE / HR:

STRENGTH:

RELAXATION

DAILY WRAP-UP

NUTRITION

CRAVINGS:

AVERSIONS:

NOTES:

MEDS / TESTS

thursday

WEIGHT ☐ PRENATAL SUPPLEMENT ☐ KEGELS ☐☐

EXERCISE

CARDIO:

RPE / HR:

STRENGTH:

RELAXATION

DAILY WRAP-UP

NUTRITION

CRAVINGS:

AVERSIONS:

NOTES:

MEDS / TESTS

DID YOU KNOW? A new baby typically results in 400 to 750 hours of lost sleep for parents in the first year. The average newborn tends to sleep for two to four hours, wake up for one to two hours, fall asleep again, and so on throughout the day.

friday

WEIGHT [ ] PRENATAL SUPPLEMENT [ ] KEGELS [|]

EXERCISE

CARDIO:

RPE / HR:

_____

_____

STRENGTH:

_____

_____

RELAXATION

DAILY WRAP-UP

NUTRITION

CRAVINGS:

_____

AVERSIONS:

_____

NOTES:

_____

_____

MEDS / TESTS

_____

_____

_____

_____

saturday

WEIGHT [ ] PRENATAL SUPPLEMENT [ ] KEGELS [|]

EXERCISE

CARDIO:

RPE / HR:

_____

_____

STRENGTH:

_____

_____

RELAXATION

DAILY WRAP-UP

NUTRITION

CRAVINGS:

_____

AVERSIONS:

_____

NOTES:

_____

_____

MEDS / TESTS

_____

_____

_____

_____

THROUGH THE AGES: Braxton Hicks contractions, false contractions common in the middle and end of pregnancy, were first described in 1872 by an English doctor named Braxton Hicks. No need to worry if you experience these: they're simply your uterus's dress rehearsal for the real thing.

sunday

WEIGHT [ ] PRENATAL SUPPLEMENT [ ] KEGELS [ ][ ]

EXERCISE

CARDIO: _____

RPE / HR: _____

_____

_____

STRENGTH: _____

_____

_____

RELAXATION

NUTRITION

CRAVINGS: _____

_____

AVERSIONS: _____

_____

NOTES: _____

_____

DAILY WRAP-UP

MEDS / TESTS

_____

_____

_____

_____

weekly wrap-up

GOALS   MET _____   EXCEEDED _____   MAYBE NEXT WEEK _____

EXERCISE   TOTAL CARDIO SESSIONS [ ]   TOTAL CARDIO HOURS [ ]   TOTAL STRENGTH SESSIONS [ ]

NOTES _____

_____

_____

NUTRITION

REFLECTIONS ON THE WEEK

week
27

Dates: _____

Goals: _____

_____

_____

monday

WEIGHT [ ]   **PRENATAL SUPPLEMENT** [ ]   KEGELS [|]

EXERCISE

CARDIO: _____

RPE / HR: _____

_____

STRENGTH: _____

_____

RELAXATION

NUTRITION

CRAVINGS: _____

AVERSIONS: _____

NOTES: _____

DAILY WRAP-UP

MEDS / TESTS

_____

_____

_____

tuesday

WEIGHT [ ]   **PRENATAL SUPPLEMENT** [ ]   KEGELS [|]

EXERCISE

CARDIO: _____

RPE / HR: _____

_____

STRENGTH: _____

_____

RELAXATION

NUTRITION

CRAVINGS: _____

AVERSIONS: _____

NOTES: _____

DAILY WRAP-UP

MEDS / TESTS

_____

_____

_____

YOUR BABY THIS WEEK: Congrats! You're beginning your third trimester. Though sounds are still a bit muted, by this point baby's hearing is sensitive enough to know your voice and the voice of other frequent visitors. Baby is getting chubby as fat deposits continue accumulating beneath the skin.

wednesday

WEIGHT ☐ PRENATAL SUPPLEMENT ☐ KEGELS ☐☐

EXERCISE

CARDIO:

RPE / HR:

STRENGTH:

RELAXATION

NUTRITION

CRAVINGS:

AVERSIONS:

NOTES:

DAILY WRAP-UP

MEDS / TESTS

thursday

WEIGHT ☐ PRENATAL SUPPLEMENT ☐ KEGELS ☐☐

EXERCISE

CARDIO:

RPE / HR:

STRENGTH:

RELAXATION

NUTRITION

CRAVINGS:

AVERSIONS:

NOTES:

DAILY WRAP-UP

MEDS / TESTS

BY THE NUMBERS: **4.1:** Number of days U.S. women stayed in the hospital after childbirth in 1970. **3.8:** Days averaged in the hospital in 1980. **2:** Days averaged in 2005 for women giving birth vaginally. **4:** Days averaged for women giving birth via Cesarean.

friday

WEIGHT ☐ PRENATAL SUPPLEMENT ☐ KEGELS ☐☐

EXERCISE

CARDIO:

RPE / HR:

STRENGTH:

RELAXATION

DAILY WRAP-UP

NUTRITION

CRAVINGS:

AVERSIONS:

NOTES:

MEDS / TESTS

saturday

WEIGHT ☐ PRENATAL SUPPLEMENT ☐ KEGELS ☐☐

EXERCISE

CARDIO:

RPE / HR:

STRENGTH:

RELAXATION

DAILY WRAP-UP

NUTRITION

CRAVINGS:

AVERSIONS:

NOTES:

MEDS / TESTS

> "Father asked us what was God's noblest work. Anna said men, but I said babies. Men are often bad; babies never are." — **LOUISA MAY ALCOTT**

sunday

WEIGHT [ ]　　PRENATAL SUPPLEMENT [ ]　　KEGELS [|]

EXERCISE

CARDIO:

RPE / HR:

STRENGTH:

RELAXATION

NUTRITION

CRAVINGS:

AVERSIONS:

NOTES:

DAILY WRAP-UP

MEDS / TESTS

weekly wrap-up

GOALS　MET _____　EXCEEDED _____　MAYBE NEXT WEEK _____

EXERCISE　TOTAL CARDIO SESSIONS [ ]　TOTAL CARDIO HOURS [ ]　TOTAL STRENGTH SESSIONS [ ]

NOTES

NUTRITION

REFLECTIONS ON THE WEEK

week
28

Dates:

Goals:

monday

WEIGHT   PRENATAL SUPPLEMENT   KEGELS

EXERCISE

CARDIO:

RPE / HR:

STRENGTH:

RELAXATION

NUTRITION

CRAVINGS:

AVERSIONS:

NOTES:

DAILY WRAP-UP

MEDS / TESTS

tuesday

WEIGHT   PRENATAL SUPPLEMENT   KEGELS

EXERCISE

CARDIO:

RPE / HR:

STRENGTH:

RELAXATION

NUTRITION

CRAVINGS:

AVERSIONS:

NOTES:

DAILY WRAP-UP

MEDS / TESTS

YOUR BABY THIS WEEK: This week your baby's brain is taking on a wrinkled and grooved appearance because of its rapid growth. Most of the lanugo has disappeared and some babies have a full head of hair by now, though being a chrome dome is normal, too.

wednesday

WEIGHT ☐ PRENATAL SUPPLEMENT ☐ KEGELS ☐☐

EXERCISE

CARDIO:

RPE / HR:

STRENGTH:

RELAXATION

NUTRITION

CRAVINGS:

AVERSIONS:

NOTES:

DAILY WRAP-UP

MEDS / TESTS

thursday

WEIGHT ☐ PRENATAL SUPPLEMENT ☐ KEGELS ☐☐

EXERCISE

CARDIO:

RPE / HR:

STRENGTH:

RELAXATION

NUTRITION

CRAVINGS:

AVERSIONS:

NOTES:

DAILY WRAP-UP

MEDS / TESTS

DID YOU KNOW? Babies play with their umbilical cord. Some experts think they give themselves a buzz by grasping it hard enough to briefly cut off their oxygen supply.

friday

WEIGHT ☐ PRENATAL SUPPLEMENT ☐ KEGELS ☐ ☐

EXERCISE

CARDIO:

RPE / HR:

STRENGTH:

RELAXATION

NUTRITION

CRAVINGS:

AVERSIONS:

NOTES:

DAILY WRAP-UP

MEDS / TESTS

saturday

WEIGHT ☐ PRENATAL SUPPLEMENT ☐ KEGELS ☐ ☐

EXERCISE

CARDIO:

RPE / HR:

STRENGTH:

RELAXATION

NUTRITION

CRAVINGS:

AVERSIONS:

NOTES:

DAILY WRAP-UP

MEDS / TESTS

THROUGH THE AGES: The youngest mother whose history is authenticated is a Peruvian girl who was 5 years, 7 months in 1939 when she delivered a 6-pound boy. In 2005, a 66-year-old Romanian woman gave birth to a girl conceived using donor eggs and donor sperm.

sunday

WEIGHT ____ PRENATAL SUPPLEMENT ____ KEGELS ____ ____

EXERCISE ____

CARDIO: ____

RPE / HR: ____

STRENGTH: ____

RELAXATION

DAILY WRAP-UP

NUTRITION ____

CRAVINGS: ____

AVERSIONS: ____

NOTES: ____

MEDS / TESTS

weekly wrap-up

GOALS   MET ____   EXCEEDED ____   MAYBE NEXT WEEK ____

EXERCISE   TOTAL CARDIO SESSIONS ____   TOTAL CARDIO HOURS ____   TOTAL STRENGTH SESSIONS ____

NOTES ____

NUTRITION

REFLECTIONS ON THE WEEK

week 29

Dates: _____
Goals: _____
_____
_____

monday

WEIGHT [ ]   PRENATAL SUPPLEMENT [ ]   KEGELS [ ][ ]

EXERCISE
CARDIO: _____
RPE / HR: _____
_____
_____
STRENGTH: _____
_____
_____

RELAXATION

NUTRITION
CRAVINGS: _____
_____
AVERSIONS: _____
NOTES: _____
_____

DAILY WRAP-UP

MEDS / TESTS
_____
_____
_____
_____

tuesday

WEIGHT [ ]   PRENATAL SUPPLEMENT [ ]   KEGELS [ ][ ]

EXERCISE
CARDIO: _____
RPE / HR: _____
_____
_____
STRENGTH: _____
_____
_____

RELAXATION

NUTRITION
CRAVINGS: _____
_____
AVERSIONS: _____
NOTES: _____
_____

DAILY WRAP-UP

MEDS / TESTS
_____
_____
_____
_____

YOUR BABY THIS WEEK: Baby's muscles and lungs are continuing to mature, and her head is growing bigger to accommodate her budding brain — which is busy growing the 100 million brain cells she'll have at birth. That's OK — by this time, mom has lost at least the same amount.

wednesday

WEIGHT ☐ PRENATAL SUPPLEMENT ☐ KEGELS ☐☐

EXERCISE

CARDIO:

RPE / HR:

STRENGTH:

RELAXATION

NUTRITION

CRAVINGS:

AVERSIONS:

NOTES:

DAILY WRAP-UP

MEDS / TESTS

thursday

WEIGHT ☐ PRENATAL SUPPLEMENT ☐ KEGELS ☐☐

EXERCISE

CARDIO:

RPE / HR:

STRENGTH:

RELAXATION

NUTRITION

CRAVINGS:

AVERSIONS:

NOTES:

DAILY WRAP-UP

MEDS / TESTS

BY THE NUMBERS: 12: Percent of women who gain 15 pounds or less during pregnancy. **25:** Percent of women who gain 16 to 25 pounds. **32:** Percent of women who gain 26 to 35 pounds. **19:** Percent of women who gain 36 to 45 pounds. **12:** Percent of women who gain 46 pounds or more.

friday

WEIGHT ☐ PRENATAL SUPPLEMENT ☐ KEGELS ☐ ☐

EXERCISE

CARDIO:

RPE / HR:

_____

_____

STRENGTH:

_____

_____

RELAXATION

NUTRITION

CRAVINGS:

_____

AVERSIONS:

_____

NOTES:

_____

DAILY WRAP-UP

MEDS / TESTS

_____

_____

_____

_____

saturday

WEIGHT ☐ PRENATAL SUPPLEMENT ☐ KEGELS ☐ ☐

EXERCISE

CARDIO:

RPE / HR:

_____

_____

STRENGTH:

_____

_____

RELAXATION

NUTRITION

CRAVINGS:

_____

AVERSIONS:

_____

NOTES:

_____

DAILY WRAP-UP

MEDS / TESTS

_____

_____

_____

_____

> "All the time we wondered and wondered who is this person coming/growing/turning/floating/swimming deep, deep inside."
> — CRESCENT DRAGONWAGON

sunday

WEIGHT ☐ PRENATAL SUPPLEMENT ☐ KEGELS ☐ ☐

EXERCISE

CARDIO: _____

RPE / HR: _____

_____

_____

STRENGTH: _____

_____

_____

RELAXATION

NUTRITION

CRAVINGS: _____

_____

AVERSIONS: _____

NOTES: _____

_____

_____

MEDS / TESTS

_____

_____

_____

_____

DAILY WRAP-UP

weekly wrap-up

GOALS   MET _____   EXCEEDED _____   MAYBE NEXT WEEK _____

EXERCISE   TOTAL CARDIO SESSIONS ☐   TOTAL CARDIO HOURS ☐   TOTAL STRENGTH SESSIONS ☐

NOTES _____

_____

_____

NUTRITION

REFLECTIONS ON THE WEEK

week
30

Dates:

Goals:

monday

WEIGHT ☐ PRENATAL SUPPLEMENT ☐ KEGELS ☐☐

EXERCISE

CARDIO:

RPE / HR:

STRENGTH:

RELAXATION

NUTRITION

CRAVINGS:

AVERSIONS:

NOTES:

DAILY WRAP-UP

MEDS / TESTS

tuesday

WEIGHT ☐ PRENATAL SUPPLEMENT ☐ KEGELS ☐☐

EXERCISE

CARDIO:

RPE / HR:

STRENGTH:

RELAXATION

NUTRITION

CRAVINGS:

AVERSIONS:

NOTES:

DAILY WRAP-UP

MEDS / TESTS

YOUR BABY THIS WEEK: You might begin to feel some uncomfortable pressure against your ribs as your baby continues to grow. She's now about 17 inches and weighs more than 3 pounds. Her eyelashes and eyebrows are fully grown, and she's plumping out.

wednesday

WEIGHT ☐ PRENATAL SUPPLEMENT ☐ KEGELS ☐☐

EXERCISE

CARDIO:

RPE / HR:

STRENGTH:

RELAXATION

NUTRITION

CRAVINGS:

AVERSIONS:

NOTES:

MEDS / TESTS

DAILY WRAP-UP

thursday

WEIGHT ☐ PRENATAL SUPPLEMENT ☐ KEGELS ☐☐

EXERCISE

CARDIO:

RPE / HR:

STRENGTH:

RELAXATION

NUTRITION

CRAVINGS:

AVERSIONS:

NOTES:

MEDS / TESTS

DAILY WRAP-UP

DID YOU KNOW? If your newborn sneezes, it doesn't mean she has a cold. It could be that her nose is runny from accumulated amniotic fluid. Chronic hiccups, the consequence of a developing respiratory system, are normal, too, and perfectly harmless.

friday

WEIGHT ☐ PRENATAL SUPPLEMENT ☐ KEGELS ☐☐

EXERCISE

CARDIO:

RPE / HR:

_____

_____

STRENGTH:

_____

_____

RELAXATION

DAILY WRAP-UP

NUTRITION

CRAVINGS:

_____

AVERSIONS:

_____

NOTES:

_____

MEDS / TESTS

_____

_____

_____

saturday

WEIGHT ☐ PRENATAL SUPPLEMENT ☐ KEGELS ☐☐

EXERCISE

CARDIO:

RPE / HR:

_____

_____

STRENGTH:

_____

DAILY WRAP-UP

RELAXATION

NUTRITION

CRAVINGS:

_____

AVERSIONS:

_____

NOTES:

_____

MEDS / TESTS

_____

_____

_____

_____

THROUGH THE AGES: A New Zealand woman holds the record for the shortest interval between two children born in separate confinements. She gave birth to a son on September 3, 1999, and then a daughter on March 30, 2000, just 208 days later.

sunday

WEIGHT [   ] PRENATAL SUPPLEMENT [   ] KEGELS [|]

EXERCISE

CARDIO: _____

RPE / HR: _____

_____

_____

STRENGTH: _____

_____

RELAXATION

NUTRITION

CRAVINGS: _____

_____

AVERSIONS: _____

_____

NOTES: _____

DAILY WRAP-UP

MEDS / TESTS

_____

_____

_____

_____

weekly wrap-up

GOALS   MET _____   EXCEEDED _____   MAYBE NEXT WEEK _____

EXERCISE   TOTAL CARDIO SESSIONS [   ]   TOTAL CARDIO HOURS [   ]   TOTAL STRENGTH SESSIONS [   ]

NOTES _____

_____

_____

NUTRITION

REFLECTIONS ON THE WEEK

week
31

Dates: _____

Goals: _____
_____
_____

monday

WEIGHT [ ]   **PRENATAL SUPPLEMENT** [ ]   **KEGELS** [ ][ ]

EXERCISE _____

CARDIO: _____

RPE / HR: _____

_____

STRENGTH: _____

_____

RELAXATION

NUTRITION _____

CRAVINGS: _____

AVERSIONS: _____

NOTES: _____

_____

DAILY WRAP-UP

MEDS / TESTS
_____
_____
_____

tuesday

WEIGHT [ ]   **PRENATAL SUPPLEMENT** [ ]   **KEGELS** [ ][ ]

EXERCISE _____

CARDIO: _____

RPE / HR: _____

_____

STRENGTH: _____

_____

RELAXATION

NUTRITION _____

CRAVINGS: _____

AVERSIONS: _____

NOTES: _____

_____

DAILY WRAP-UP

MEDS / TESTS
_____
_____
_____

YOUR BABY THIS WEEK: By now, baby is flushing out several cups of urine a day from her body into the amniotic fluid and swallowing the fluid, which is completely replaced several times a day. Baby has assumed the fetal position because there's no room for her legs to straighten out.

wednesday

WEIGHT ☐　　PRENATAL SUPPLEMENT ☐　　KEGELS ☐☐

EXERCISE

CARDIO: _____

RPE / HR: _____

_____

_____

STRENGTH: _____

_____

_____

RELAXATION

DAILY WRAP-UP

NUTRITION

CRAVINGS: _____

_____

AVERSIONS: _____

_____

NOTES: _____

_____

MEDS / TESTS

_____

_____

_____

_____

thursday

WEIGHT ☐　　PRENATAL SUPPLEMENT ☐　　KEGELS ☐☐

EXERCISE

CARDIO: _____

RPE / HR: _____

_____

_____

STRENGTH: _____

_____

_____

RELAXATION

DAILY WRAP-UP

NUTRITION

CRAVINGS: _____

_____

AVERSIONS: _____

_____

NOTES: _____

_____

MEDS / TESTS

_____

_____

_____

_____

BY THE NUMBERS: 22 pounds, 8 ounces: Weight of heaviest baby born to a healthy mother, in Italy in 1955, according to the <u>Guinness Book of World Records</u>. **7.5 pounds:** Weight of average newborn. **10 ounces:** Weight of smallest known surviving newborn, delivered in 2007 at 21 weeks, 6 days.

friday

WEIGHT | PRENATAL SUPPLEMENT | KEGELS

EXERCISE

CARDIO:

RPE / HR:

STRENGTH:

RELAXATION

NUTRITION

CRAVINGS:

AVERSIONS:

NOTES:

DAILY WRAP-UP

MEDS / TESTS

saturday

WEIGHT | PRENATAL SUPPLEMENT | KEGELS

EXERCISE

CARDIO:

RPE / HR:

STRENGTH:

RELAXATION

NUTRITION

CRAVINGS:

AVERSIONS:

NOTES:

DAILY WRAP-UP

MEDS / TESTS

> "Loving a baby is a circular business, a kind of feedback loop. The more you give, the more you get, and the more you get, the more you feel like giving."
> — **PENELOPE LEACH**, author of <u>Your Baby and Child: From Birth to Age Five</u>

sunday

WEIGHT ___ PRENATAL SUPPLEMENT ___ KEGELS ___ ___

EXERCISE

CARDIO:

RPE / HR:

STRENGTH:

RELAXATION

DAILY WRAP-UP

NUTRITION

CRAVINGS:

AVERSIONS:

NOTES:

MEDS / TESTS

weekly wrap-up

GOALS MET _____ EXCEEDED _____ MAYBE NEXT WEEK _____

EXERCISE TOTAL CARDIO SESSIONS ___ TOTAL CARDIO HOURS ___ TOTAL STRENGTH SESSIONS ___

NOTES

NUTRITION

REFLECTIONS ON THE WEEK

week
32

Dates: _____

Goals: _____

_____

_____

monday

WEIGHT ☐   PRENATAL SUPPLEMENT ☐   KEGELS ☐☐

EXERCISE

CARDIO: _____

RPE / HR: _____

_____

_____

STRENGTH: _____

_____

_____

RELAXATION

DAILY WRAP-UP

NUTRITION

CRAVINGS: _____

AVERSIONS: _____

NOTES: _____

_____

MEDS / TESTS

_____

_____

_____

_____

tuesday

WEIGHT ☐   PRENATAL SUPPLEMENT ☐   KEGELS ☐☐

EXERCISE

CARDIO: _____

RPE / HR: _____

_____

_____

STRENGTH: _____

_____

_____

RELAXATION

DAILY WRAP-UP

NUTRITION

CRAVINGS: _____

AVERSIONS: _____

NOTES: _____

_____

MEDS / TESTS

_____

_____

_____

YOUR BABY THIS WEEK: When you feel powerful kicks under your rib cage and the hard ball of the baby's head pressing down on your bladder, you'll know she's inverted to a head-down position. If not, there's a good chance she will turn in the coming weeks. Baby sleeps about 70 percent of the time.

wednesday

WEIGHT ☐   PRENATAL SUPPLEMENT ☐   KEGELS ☐☐

EXERCISE

CARDIO:

RPE / HR:

STRENGTH:

RELAXATION

NUTRITION

CRAVINGS:

AVERSIONS:

NOTES:

DAILY WRAP-UP

MEDS / TESTS

thursday

WEIGHT ☐   PRENATAL SUPPLEMENT ☐   KEGELS ☐☐

EXERCISE

CARDIO:

RPE / HR:

STRENGTH:

RELAXATION

NUTRITION

CRAVINGS:

AVERSIONS:

NOTES:

DAILY WRAP-UP

MEDS / TESTS

DID YOU KNOW? Ultrasound scans often catch babies smiling in the last few weeks before they are born. Birth seems to interrupt their good mood, though, and they may not smile again for the first twelve weeks of life. If you see babies smile before that, it's probably because they're passing gas.

friday

WEIGHT ☐ PRENATAL SUPPLEMENT ☐ KEGELS ☐☐

EXERCISE

CARDIO:

RPE / HR:

STRENGTH:

RELAXATION

NUTRITION

CRAVINGS:

AVERSIONS:

NOTES:

MEDS / TESTS

DAILY WRAP-UP

saturday

WEIGHT ☐ PRENATAL SUPPLEMENT ☐ KEGELS ☐☐

EXERCISE

CARDIO:

RPE / HR:

STRENGTH:

RELAXATION

NUTRITION

CRAVINGS:

AVERSIONS:

NOTES:

MEDS / TESTS

DAILY WRAP-UP

THROUGH THE AGES: The first successful birth from frozen sperm occurred in 1954; it was another 30 years before the first baby was born from a frozen embryo. The first confirmed birth using frozen eggs occurred in 1996, and in 2000, twins conceived from both frozen eggs and frozen sperm were born.

sunday

WEIGHT [   ]   PRENATAL SUPPLEMENT [   ]   KEGELS [|]

EXERCISE

CARDIO:

RPE / HR:

STRENGTH:

RELAXATION

NUTRITION

CRAVINGS:

AVERSIONS:

NOTES:

MEDS / TESTS

DAILY WRAP-UP

weekly wrap-up

GOALS   MET _____   EXCEEDED _____   MAYBE NEXT WEEK _____

EXERCISE   TOTAL CARDIO SESSIONS [   ]   TOTAL CARDIO HOURS [   ]   TOTAL STRENGTH SESSIONS [   ]

NOTES

NUTRITION

REFLECTIONS ON THE WEEK

week

33

Dates: _____

Goals: _____

_____

_____

mon∂ay

WEIGHT ☐ **PRENATAL SUPPLEMENT** ☐ KEGELS ☐☐

EXERCISE

CARDIO: _____

RPE / HR: _____

_____

_____

STRENGTH: _____

_____

_____

RELAXATION

DAILY WRAP-UP

NUTRITION

CRAVINGS: _____

_____

AVERSIONS: _____

_____

NOTES: _____

_____

MEDS / TESTS

_____

_____

_____

_____

tues∂ay

WEIGHT ☐ **PRENATAL SUPPLEMENT** ☐ KEGELS ☐☐

EXERCISE

CARDIO: _____

RPE / HR: _____

_____

_____

STRENGTH: _____

_____

_____

RELAXATION

DAILY WRAP-UP

NUTRITION

CRAVINGS: _____

_____

AVERSIONS: _____

_____

NOTES: _____

_____

MEDS / TESTS

_____

_____

_____

_____

YOUR BABY THIS WEEK: Your baby is now doing some serious packing for labor and delivery — as in packing on the pounds. You'll be gaining about a pound a week from here on, mostly due to the baby's weight gain. Baby weighs about 4½ pounds and is 17 inches long, with completely grown toenails.

wednesday

WEIGHT ☐   PRENATAL SUPPLEMENT ☐   KEGELS ☐☐

EXERCISE

CARDIO:

RPE / HR:

STRENGTH:

RELAXATION

NUTRITION

CRAVINGS:

AVERSIONS:

NOTES:

MEDS / TESTS

DAILY WRAP-UP

thursday

WEIGHT ☐   PRENATAL SUPPLEMENT ☐   KEGELS ☐☐

EXERCISE

CARDIO:

RPE / HR:

STRENGTH:

RELAXATION

NUTRITION

CRAVINGS:

AVERSIONS:

NOTES:

MEDS / TESTS

DAILY WRAP-UP

BY THE NUMBERS: 12,500: The average number of births on any given Tuesday, the most popular day of the week for babies to make their entrance. **8,300:** Number of births on Sunday, the slowest day of the week for births, largely because doctors don't schedule C-sections and inductions on weekends.

friday

WEIGHT ☐   PRENATAL SUPPLEMENT ☐   KEGELS ☐☐

EXERCISE

CARDIO:

RPE / HR:

STRENGTH:

RELAXATION

NUTRITION

CRAVINGS:

AVERSIONS:

NOTES:

MEDS / TESTS

DAILY WRAP-UP

saturday

WEIGHT ☐   PRENATAL SUPPLEMENT ☐   KEGELS ☐☐

EXERCISE

CARDIO:

RPE / HR:

STRENGTH:

RELAXATION

NUTRITION

CRAVINGS:

AVERSIONS:

NOTES:

MEDS / TESTS

DAILY WRAP-UP

"Think of stretch marks as pregnancy service stripes." —JOYCE ARMOR

sunday

WEIGHT [   ] PRENATAL SUPPLEMENT [   ] KEGELS [|]

EXERCISE

CARDIO:

RPE / HR:

STRENGTH:

RELAXATION

DAILY WRAP-UP

NUTRITION

CRAVINGS:

AVERSIONS:

NOTES:

MEDS / TESTS

weekly wrap-up

GOALS   MET _____   EXCEEDED _____   MAYBE NEXT WEEK _____

EXERCISE   TOTAL CARDIO SESSIONS [   ]   TOTAL CARDIO HOURS [   ]   TOTAL STRENGTH SESSIONS [   ]

NOTES

NUTRITION

REFLECTIONS ON THE WEEK

week
34

Dates: _____

Goals: _____

_____

_____

monday

WEIGHT [ ] **PRENATAL SUPPLEMENT** [ ] KEGELS [|]

EXERCISE

CARDIO: _____

RPE / HR: _____

_____

_____

STRENGTH: _____

_____

_____

RELAXATION

DAILY WRAP-UP

NUTRITION

CRAVINGS: _____

AVERSIONS: _____

NOTES: _____

_____

MEDS / TESTS

_____

_____

_____

_____

tuesday

WEIGHT [ ] **PRENATAL SUPPLEMENT** [ ] KEGELS [|]

EXERCISE

CARDIO: _____

RPE / HR: _____

_____

_____

STRENGTH: _____

_____

_____

RELAXATION

DAILY WRAP-UP

NUTRITION

CRAVINGS: _____

AVERSIONS: _____

NOTES: _____

_____

MEDS / TESTS

_____

_____

_____

_____

YOUR BABY THIS WEEK: At this point, 99 percent of babies can survive outside the womb. A Caucasian baby's eyes are usually blue now, regardless of the final color they will become. Final formation of eye pigmentation generally requires a few weeks' exposure to light but can change even moments after birth.

wednesday

WEIGHT ☐ PRENATAL SUPPLEMENT ☐ KEGELS ☐☐

EXERCISE

CARDIO:

RPE / HR:

STRENGTH:

RELAXATION

NUTRITION

CRAVINGS:

AVERSIONS:

NOTES:

DAILY WRAP-UP

MEDS / TESTS

thursday

WEIGHT ☐ PRENATAL SUPPLEMENT ☐ KEGELS ☐☐

EXERCISE

CARDIO:

RPE / HR:

STRENGTH:

RELAXATION

NUTRITION

CRAVINGS:

AVERSIONS:

NOTES:

DAILY WRAP-UP

MEDS / TESTS

DID YOU KNOW? Babies don't have kneecaps when they are born. They develop only during the latter half of the first year.

friday

WEIGHT | PRENATAL SUPPLEMENT | KEGELS

EXERCISE

CARDIO:

RPE / HR:

STRENGTH:

RELAXATION

NUTRITION

CRAVINGS:

AVERSIONS:

NOTES:

DAILY WRAP-UP

MEDS / TESTS

saturday

WEIGHT | PRENATAL SUPPLEMENT | KEGELS

EXERCISE

CARDIO:

RPE / HR:

STRENGTH:

RELAXATION

NUTRITION

CRAVINGS:

AVERSIONS:

NOTES:

DAILY WRAP-UP

MEDS / TESTS

THROUGH THE AGES: Many women in India, Taiwan, and China are confined to bed rest for four to six weeks following childbirth, an ancient tradition. Even as recently as the early twentieth century, many American women were hospitalized for up to six weeks — with the first two spent on bed rest.

sunday

WEIGHT ☐   PRENATAL SUPPLEMENT ☐   KEGELS ☐ ☐

EXERCISE

CARDIO:

RPE / HR:

STRENGTH:

RELAXATION

NUTRITION

CRAVINGS:

AVERSIONS:

NOTES:

DAILY WRAP-UP

MEDS / TESTS

weekly wrap-up

GOALS   MET _____   EXCEEDED _____   MAYBE NEXT WEEK _____

EXERCISE   TOTAL CARDIO SESSIONS ☐   TOTAL CARDIO HOURS ☐   TOTAL STRENGTH SESSIONS ☐

NOTES

NUTRITION

REFLECTIONS ON THE WEEK

week
35

Dates: _____

Goals: _____
_____
_____

monday

WEIGHT [ ]   **PRENATAL SUPPLEMENT** [ ]   KEGELS [|]

EXERCISE

CARDIO: _____

RPE / HR: _____

_____

_____

STRENGTH: _____

_____

_____

RELAXATION

NUTRITION

CRAVINGS: _____

_____

AVERSIONS: _____

_____

NOTES: _____

_____

DAILY WRAP-UP

MEDS / TESTS

_____

_____

_____

_____

tuesday

WEIGHT [ ]   **PRENATAL SUPPLEMENT** [ ]   KEGELS [|]

EXERCISE

CARDIO: _____

RPE / HR: _____

_____

_____

STRENGTH: _____

_____

_____

RELAXATION

NUTRITION

CRAVINGS: _____

_____

AVERSIONS: _____

_____

NOTES: _____

_____

DAILY WRAP-UP

MEDS / TESTS

_____

_____

_____

_____

YOUR BABY THIS WEEK: By now you'll feel bouncing in your belly as baby develops sleeping patterns that unfortunately have little to do with day and night. Most of baby's physical development is now complete; she'll spend the next few weeks putting on weight.

wednesday

WEIGHT ☐ PRENATAL SUPPLEMENT ☐ KEGELS ☐☐

EXERCISE

CARDIO:

RPE / HR:

STRENGTH:

RELAXATION

NUTRITION

CRAVINGS:

AVERSIONS:

NOTES:

DAILY WRAP-UP

MEDS / TESTS

thursday

WEIGHT ☐ PRENATAL SUPPLEMENT ☐ KEGELS ☐☐

EXERCISE

CARDIO:

RPE / HR:

STRENGTH:

RELAXATION

NUTRITION

CRAVINGS:

AVERSIONS:

NOTES:

DAILY WRAP-UP

MEDS / TESTS

BY THE NUMBERS: **15:** Percent of newborn's weight that is body fat. **80:** Percent of baby's body fat located directly under surface of baby's skin. **20:** Percent found on organs and muscle tissue. **12 to 20:** Typical percent of body fat of healthy adult males. **16 to 26:** Typical percent of body fat of healthy women.

friday

WEIGHT ☐ PRENATAL SUPPLEMENT ☐ KEGELS ☐☐

EXERCISE

CARDIO:

RPE / HR:

STRENGTH:

RELAXATION

DAILY WRAP-UP

NUTRITION

CRAVINGS:

AVERSIONS:

NOTES:

MEDS / TESTS

saturday

WEIGHT ☐ PRENATAL SUPPLEMENT ☐ KEGELS ☐☐

EXERCISE

CARDIO:

RPE / HR:

STRENGTH:

RELAXATION

DAILY WRAP-UP

NUTRITION

CRAVINGS:

AVERSIONS:

NOTES:

MEDS / TESTS

> "We never know the love of the parent till we become parents ourselves."
> — HENRY WARD BEECHER

sunday

WEIGHT ☐ PRENATAL SUPPLEMENT ☐ KEGELS ☐☐

EXERCISE

CARDIO:

RPE / HR:

STRENGTH:

RELAXATION

NUTRITION

CRAVINGS:

AVERSIONS:

NOTES:

MEDS / TESTS

DAILY WRAP-UP

weekly wrap-up

GOALS   MET _____   EXCEEDED _____   MAYBE NEXT WEEK _____

EXERCISE   TOTAL CARDIO SESSIONS ☐   TOTAL CARDIO HOURS ☐   TOTAL STRENGTH SESSIONS ☐

NOTES

NUTRITION

REFLECTIONS ON THE WEEK

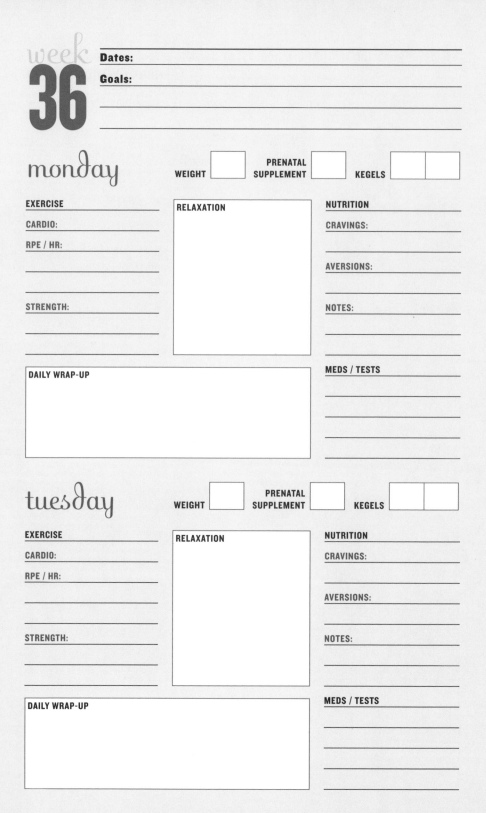

week 36

Dates: _____

Goals: _____
_____
_____

monday

WEIGHT ☐ PRENATAL SUPPLEMENT ☐ KEGELS ☐☐

EXERCISE

CARDIO: _____

RPE / HR: _____
_____
_____

STRENGTH: _____
_____
_____

RELAXATION

DAILY WRAP-UP

NUTRITION

CRAVINGS: _____

AVERSIONS: _____

NOTES: _____
_____

MEDS / TESTS
_____
_____
_____
_____

tuesday

WEIGHT ☐ PRENATAL SUPPLEMENT ☐ KEGELS ☐☐

EXERCISE

CARDIO: _____

RPE / HR: _____
_____
_____

STRENGTH: _____
_____
_____

RELAXATION

DAILY WRAP-UP

NUTRITION

CRAVINGS: _____

AVERSIONS: _____

NOTES: _____

MEDS / TESTS
_____
_____
_____

YOUR BABY THIS WEEK: Baby is surrounded by the maximum amount of amniotic fluid, so it's really getting crowded in there. With fat continuing to deposit, baby is starting to dimple at the elbows and knees, and those neck folds and wrist folds are developing.

wednesday

WEIGHT ☐   PRENATAL SUPPLEMENT ☐   KEGELS ☐ ☐

EXERCISE

CARDIO:

RPE / HR:

STRENGTH:

RELAXATION

NUTRITION

CRAVINGS:

AVERSIONS:

NOTES:

DAILY WRAP-UP

MEDS / TESTS

thursday

WEIGHT ☐   PRENATAL SUPPLEMENT ☐   KEGELS ☐ ☐

EXERCISE

CARDIO:

RPE / HR:

STRENGTH:

RELAXATION

NUTRITION

CRAVINGS:

AVERSIONS:

NOTES:

DAILY WRAP-UP

MEDS / TESTS

DID YOU KNOW? Newborns have skin that is thinner and contains a higher moisture content than an adult's. They also have less melanin (skin pigmentation) than older children and adults, so their skin is even more susceptible to sun damage.

friday

WEIGHT ☐ PRENATAL SUPPLEMENT ☐ KEGELS ☐☐

EXERCISE

CARDIO:

RPE / HR:

STRENGTH:

RELAXATION

NUTRITION

CRAVINGS:

AVERSIONS:

NOTES:

DAILY WRAP-UP

MEDS / TESTS

saturday

WEIGHT ☐ PRENATAL SUPPLEMENT ☐ KEGELS ☐☐

EXERCISE

CARDIO:

RPE / HR:

STRENGTH:

RELAXATION

NUTRITION

CRAVINGS:

AVERSIONS:

NOTES:

DAILY WRAP-UP

MEDS / TESTS

THROUGH THE AGES: A nineteenth-century Russian custom was for the midwife to require the laboring woman and her husband to name anyone besides their spouse with whom they'd had sex. If the labor was easy, it was believed all had told the truth; if labor was difficult, someone had lied.

sunday

WEIGHT ☐ PRENATAL SUPPLEMENT ☐ KEGELS ☐☐

EXERCISE _____

CARDIO: _____

RPE / HR: _____

_____

_____

STRENGTH: _____

_____

_____

RELAXATION

DAILY WRAP-UP

NUTRITION _____

CRAVINGS: _____

_____

AVERSIONS: _____

_____

NOTES: _____

_____

MEDS / TESTS

_____

_____

_____

_____

weekly wrap-up

GOALS   MET _____   EXCEEDED _____   MAYBE NEXT WEEK _____

EXERCISE   TOTAL CARDIO SESSIONS ☐   TOTAL CARDIO HOURS ☐   TOTAL STRENGTH SESSIONS ☐

NOTES _____

_____

_____

NUTRITION

REFLECTIONS ON THE WEEK

week 37

Dates: _____

Goals: _____
_____
_____
_____

monday

WEIGHT [ ] **PRENATAL SUPPLEMENT** [ ] **KEGELS** [ ][ ]

EXERCISE

CARDIO: _____

RPE / HR: _____

_____

STRENGTH: _____

_____

RELAXATION

DAILY WRAP-UP

NUTRITION

CRAVINGS: _____

AVERSIONS: _____

NOTES: _____

MEDS / TESTS

_____
_____
_____
_____

tuesday

WEIGHT [ ] **PRENATAL SUPPLEMENT** [ ] **KEGELS** [ ][ ]

EXERCISE

CARDIO: _____

RPE / HR: _____

_____

STRENGTH: _____

_____

RELAXATION

DAILY WRAP-UP

NUTRITION

CRAVINGS: _____

AVERSIONS: _____

NOTES: _____

MEDS / TESTS

_____
_____
_____
_____

YOUR BABY THIS WEEK: If you're breathing easier these days, it's because baby's head has probably dropped, taking the pressure off your rib cage and lungs. At this point, she's considered full term and could be born safely at anytime. She's likely at least 6 pounds and close to 20 inches.

wednesday

WEIGHT ☐ PRENATAL SUPPLEMENT ☐ KEGELS ☐☐

EXERCISE

CARDIO:

RPE / HR:

STRENGTH:

RELAXATION

NUTRITION

CRAVINGS:

AVERSIONS:

NOTES:

DAILY WRAP-UP

MEDS / TESTS

thursday

WEIGHT ☐ PRENATAL SUPPLEMENT ☐ KEGELS ☐☐

EXERCISE

CARDIO:

RPE / HR:

STRENGTH:

RELAXATION

NUTRITION

CRAVINGS:

AVERSIONS:

NOTES:

DAILY WRAP-UP

MEDS / TESTS

BY THE NUMBERS: **2:** Average length, in feet, of newborn's umbilical cord. **¾:** Diameter, in inches, of typical umbilical cord at birth. **4:** Speed, in MPH, that the bloodstream travels in the umbilical cord. **30:** Number of seconds it takes for blood to complete the roundtrip through the cord and the baby.

friday

WEIGHT [ ] PRENATAL SUPPLEMENT [ ] KEGELS [ ][ ]

EXERCISE

CARDIO:

RPE / HR:

STRENGTH:

RELAXATION

NUTRITION

CRAVINGS:

AVERSIONS:

NOTES:

DAILY WRAP-UP

MEDS / TESTS

saturday

WEIGHT [ ] PRENATAL SUPPLEMENT [ ] KEGELS [ ][ ]

EXERCISE

CARDIO:

RPE / HR:

STRENGTH:

RELAXATION

NUTRITION

CRAVINGS:

AVERSIONS:

NOTES:

DAILY WRAP-UP

MEDS / TESTS

"Pay attention to the pregnant woman! There is no one more important than she." — Saying among the Chagga tribe of Tanzania

sunday

WEIGHT ☐ PRENATAL SUPPLEMENT ☐ KEGELS ☐ ☐

EXERCISE

CARDIO:

RPE / HR:

STRENGTH:

RELAXATION

NUTRITION

CRAVINGS:

AVERSIONS:

NOTES:

MEDS / TESTS

DAILY WRAP-UP

weekly wrap-up

GOALS MET _____ EXCEEDED _____ MAYBE NEXT WEEK _____

EXERCISE TOTAL CARDIO SESSIONS ☐ TOTAL CARDIO HOURS ☐ TOTAL STRENGTH SESSIONS ☐

NOTES

NUTRITION

REFLECTIONS ON THE WEEK

week
38

Dates: _____

Goals: _____

_____

_____

_____

monday

WEIGHT ☐ PRENATAL SUPPLEMENT ☐ KEGELS ☐☐

EXERCISE

CARDIO: _____

RPE / HR: _____

_____

_____

STRENGTH: _____

_____

_____

RELAXATION

DAILY WRAP-UP

NUTRITION

CRAVINGS: _____

AVERSIONS: _____

NOTES: _____

_____

MEDS / TESTS

_____

_____

_____

_____

tuesday

WEIGHT ☐ PRENATAL SUPPLEMENT ☐ KEGELS ☐☐

EXERCISE

CARDIO: _____

RPE / HR: _____

_____

_____

STRENGTH: _____

_____

_____

RELAXATION

DAILY WRAP-UP

NUTRITION

CRAVINGS: _____

AVERSIONS: _____

NOTES: _____

MEDS / TESTS

_____

_____

_____

_____

YOUR BABY THIS WEEK: Yucky but necessary: meconium, a greenish black substance that constitutes your baby's first bowel movement, is beginning to accumulate. It's formed by baby sucking and swallowing amniotic fluid and shedding cells from the intestines, skin, and lanugo hair.

wednesday

WEIGHT ☐   PRENATAL SUPPLEMENT ☐   KEGELS ☐☐

EXERCISE

CARDIO:

RPE / HR:

STRENGTH:

RELAXATION

NUTRITION

CRAVINGS:

AVERSIONS:

NOTES:

DAILY WRAP-UP

MEDS / TESTS

thursday

WEIGHT ☐   PRENATAL SUPPLEMENT ☐   KEGELS ☐☐

EXERCISE

CARDIO:

RPE / HR:

STRENGTH:

RELAXATION

NUTRITION

CRAVINGS:

AVERSIONS:

NOTES:

DAILY WRAP-UP

MEDS / TESTS

DID YOU KNOW? Babies can't talk when they're born because their voice box is not developed, but they immediately start practicing the lip and tongue movements necessary to form words. When they actually do begin to talk, babies probably know 100 words without being able to say a single one.

friday

WEIGHT ☐   PRENATAL SUPPLEMENT ☐   KEGELS ☐☐

EXERCISE

CARDIO:

RPE / HR:

STRENGTH:

RELAXATION

NUTRITION

CRAVINGS:

AVERSIONS:

NOTES:

DAILY WRAP-UP

MEDS / TESTS

saturday

WEIGHT ☐   PRENATAL SUPPLEMENT ☐   KEGELS ☐☐

EXERCISE

CARDIO:

RPE / HR:

STRENGTH:

RELAXATION

NUTRITION

CRAVINGS:

AVERSIONS:

NOTES:

DAILY WRAP-UP

MEDS / TESTS

THROUGH THE AGES: When a baby was born to an ancient Greek family, a naked father carried his child, in a ritual dance, around the household. Children of wealthy families were dipped in olive oil at birth to keep them hairless throughout their lives, apparently a prized trait among the Greeks.

sunday

WEIGHT ☐   PRENATAL SUPPLEMENT ☐   KEGELS ☐☐

EXERCISE

CARDIO:

RPE / HR:

STRENGTH:

RELAXATION

NUTRITION

CRAVINGS:

AVERSIONS:

NOTES:

MEDS / TESTS

DAILY WRAP-UP

weekly wrap-up

GOALS   MET _____   EXCEEDED _____   MAYBE NEXT WEEK _____

EXERCISE   TOTAL CARDIO SESSIONS ☐   TOTAL CARDIO HOURS ☐   TOTAL STRENGTH SESSIONS ☐

NOTES _____

NUTRITION

REFLECTIONS ON THE WEEK

week 39

Dates: _____

Goals: _____

_____

_____

monday

WEIGHT [ ]   PRENATAL SUPPLEMENT [ ]   KEGELS [|]

EXERCISE

CARDIO: _____

RPE / HR: _____

_____

STRENGTH: _____

_____

_____

RELAXATION

DAILY WRAP-UP

NUTRITION

CRAVINGS: _____

_____

AVERSIONS: _____

_____

NOTES: _____

_____

MEDS / TESTS

_____

_____

_____

_____

tuesday

WEIGHT [ ]   PRENATAL SUPPLEMENT [ ]   KEGELS [|]

EXERCISE

CARDIO: _____

RPE / HR: _____

_____

STRENGTH: _____

_____

RELAXATION

DAILY WRAP-UP

NUTRITION

CRAVINGS: _____

_____

AVERSIONS: _____

_____

NOTES: _____

_____

MEDS / TESTS

_____

_____

_____

_____

YOUR BABY THIS WEEK: Are you ready? Your baby nearly is! She's likely to weigh at least 7 pounds by now, and she'll continue to fatten up in order to help control body temperature after birth. Baby's body has grown enough to catch up with her head, which has the same circumference as her abdomen.

wednesday

WEIGHT ☐   PRENATAL SUPPLEMENT ☐   KEGELS ☐☐

EXERCISE

CARDIO:

RPE / HR:

STRENGTH:

RELAXATION

DAILY WRAP-UP

NUTRITION

CRAVINGS:

AVERSIONS:

NOTES:

MEDS / TESTS

thursday

WEIGHT ☐   PRENATAL SUPPLEMENT ☐   KEGELS ☐☐

EXERCISE

CARDIO:

RPE / HR:

STRENGTH:

RELAXATION

DAILY WRAP-UP

NUTRITION

CRAVINGS:

AVERSIONS:

NOTES:

MEDS / TESTS

BY THE NUMBERS: **1 to 1.5:** Weight, in pounds, that each breast gains during pregnancy in preparation for nursing. **2:** Number of hours it takes for milk-producing cells of the breasts to manufacture enough milk for the next feeding. **500 to 650:** Number of calories per day that milk production burns.

friday

WEIGHT ☐   **PRENATAL SUPPLEMENT** ☐   KEGELS ☐☐

EXERCISE

CARDIO:

RPE / HR:

STRENGTH:

RELAXATION

NUTRITION

CRAVINGS:

AVERSIONS:

NOTES:

DAILY WRAP-UP

MEDS / TESTS

saturday

WEIGHT ☐   **PRENATAL SUPPLEMENT** ☐   KEGELS ☐☐

EXERCISE

CARDIO:

RPE / HR:

STRENGTH:

RELAXATION

NUTRITION

CRAVINGS:

AVERSIONS:

NOTES:

DAILY WRAP-UP

MEDS / TESTS

> "Making the decision to have a child — it's momentous. It is to decide forever to have your heart go walking around outside your body."
> — ELIZABETH STONE, nineteenth-century writer

sunday

WEIGHT ☐ PRENATAL SUPPLEMENT ☐ KEGELS ☐☐

EXERCISE

CARDIO:

RPE / HR:

STRENGTH:

RELAXATION

NUTRITION

CRAVINGS:

AVERSIONS:

NOTES:

DAILY WRAP-UP

MEDS / TESTS

weekly wrap-up

GOALS   MET _____   EXCEEDED _____   MAYBE NEXT WEEK _____

EXERCISE   TOTAL CARDIO SESSIONS ☐   TOTAL CARDIO HOURS ☐   TOTAL STRENGTH SESSIONS ☐

NOTES

NUTRITION

REFLECTIONS ON THE WEEK

week
40

Dates:

Goals:

monday

WEIGHT ☐ **PRENATAL SUPPLEMENT** ☐ **KEGELS** ☐ ☐

EXERCISE

CARDIO:

RPE / HR:

STRENGTH:

RELAXATION

NUTRITION

CRAVINGS:

AVERSIONS:

NOTES:

DAILY WRAP-UP

MEDS / TESTS

tuesday

WEIGHT ☐ **PRENATAL SUPPLEMENT** ☐ **KEGELS** ☐ ☐

EXERCISE

CARDIO:

RPE / HR:

STRENGTH:

RELAXATION

NUTRITION

CRAVINGS:

AVERSIONS:

NOTES:

DAILY WRAP-UP

MEDS / TESTS

YOUR BABY THIS WEEK: Your little pumpkin is now fully cooked —
about 15 percent body fat — and ready to greet the world. Get ready to meet a
person who will bring you great joy and forever change life as you know it.

wednesday

WEIGHT [ ] PRENATAL SUPPLEMENT [ ] KEGELS [ ][ ]

EXERCISE

CARDIO:

RPE / HR:

STRENGTH:

RELAXATION

NUTRITION

CRAVINGS:

AVERSIONS:

NOTES:

DAILY WRAP-UP

MEDS / TESTS

thursday

WEIGHT [ ] PRENATAL SUPPLEMENT [ ] KEGELS [ ][ ]

EXERCISE

CARDIO:

RPE / HR:

STRENGTH:

RELAXATION

NUTRITION

CRAVINGS:

AVERSIONS:

NOTES:

DAILY WRAP-UP

MEDS / TESTS

DID YOU KNOW? Nearly all mothers carry their newborn on their left side the majority of the time so that baby's head is next to mother's heart. Hearing a mother's heartbeat soothes a baby. Most new moms also instinctively rock their babe at the same pace as their heart rate.

friday

WEIGHT ☐ PRENATAL SUPPLEMENT ☐ KEGELS ☐☐

EXERCISE

CARDIO:

RPE / HR:

STRENGTH:

RELAXATION

DAILY WRAP-UP

NUTRITION

CRAVINGS:

AVERSIONS:

NOTES:

MEDS / TESTS

saturday

WEIGHT ☐ PRENATAL SUPPLEMENT ☐ KEGELS ☐☐

EXERCISE

CARDIO:

RPE / HR:

STRENGTH:

RELAXATION

DAILY WRAP-UP

NUTRITION

CRAVINGS:

AVERSIONS:

NOTES:

MEDS / TESTS

THROUGH THE AGES: The first Mother's Day observance took place in 1908. In 1914, Congress passed legislation designating the second Sunday in May as Mother's Day. Each year, more than $5 billion worth of Mother's Day greeting cards are sold.

sunday

WEIGHT ☐ PRENATAL SUPPLEMENT ☐ KEGELS ☐☐

EXERCISE

CARDIO:

RPE / HR:

STRENGTH:

RELAXATION

NUTRITION

CRAVINGS:

AVERSIONS:

NOTES:

DAILY WRAP-UP

MEDS / TESTS

weekly wrap-up

GOALS MET _____ EXCEEDED _____ MAYBE NEXT WEEK _____

EXERCISE TOTAL CARDIO SESSIONS ☐ TOTAL CARDIO HOURS ☐ TOTAL STRENGTH SESSIONS ☐

NOTES

NUTRITION

REFLECTIONS ON THE WEEK

Prenatal Records

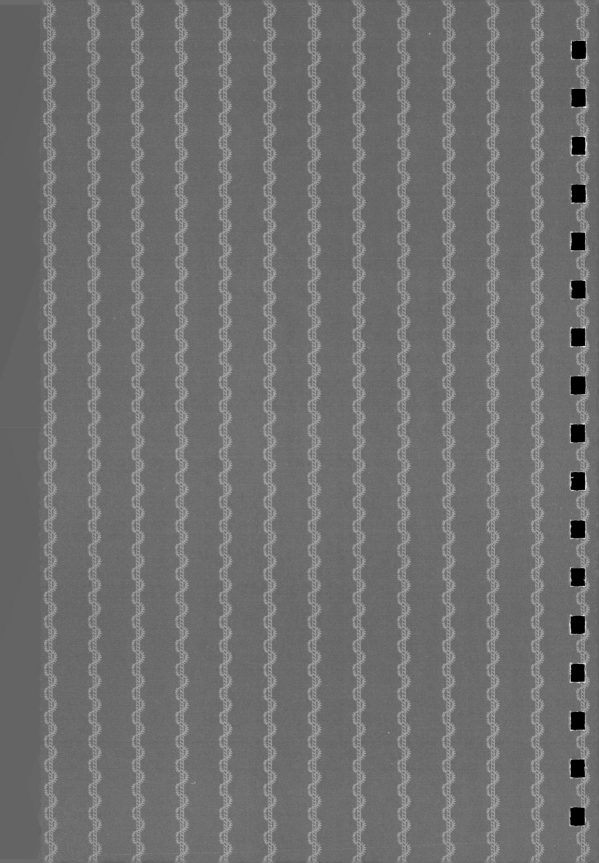

Prenatal Care Records

PRENATAL CHECKUP RECORD

Pregnancy can make you feel like you've been turned into a science experiment for your healthcare provider. You're poked, prodded, tested, weighed, measured, photographed, and studied more closely than the frog you dissected in tenth-grade biology class. Just tell yourself it's worth the trouble and discomfort because it's all for the good of the baby. Once you hold your little peanut in your arms, you'll forget the nurse who confused your blood draw with a game of darts.

Naturally, your doctor will record all of the information below—and then some—so it's hardly essential to document the data yourself. Still, many women find it fascinating to chart the changes in their bodies. Even if you're not inclined to record your urinalysis results or your little one's heart rate, it's a good idea to jot down your questions for the doctor before each appointment. You might get so enthralled gazing at your baby via the ultrasound that you completely forget to ask if leaky nipples are normal or if it's OK to drink a diet soda once in a while. Likewise, while you're still in the examining room, note any new advice or instructions your health practitioner has to offer.

Checkup 1

DATE/TIME:

QUESTIONS TO ASK:

PRACTITIONER ADVICE/INSTRUCTIONS:

BLOOD PRESSURE: PULSE:

URINALYSIS: SUGAR: PROTEIN:

FUNDAL HEIGHT: FETAL HEART RATE:

BLOOD TEST RESULTS:

Checkup 2

DATE/TIME:

QUESTIONS TO ASK:

PRACTITIONER ADVICE/INSTRUCTIONS:

BLOOD PRESSURE: PULSE:

URINALYSIS: SUGAR: PROTEIN:

FUNDAL HEIGHT: FETAL HEART RATE:

BLOOD TEST RESULTS:

Checkup 3

DATE/TIME:

QUESTIONS TO ASK:

PRACTITIONER ADVICE/INSTRUCTIONS:

BLOOD PRESSURE: PULSE:

URINALYSIS: SUGAR: PROTEIN:

FUNDAL HEIGHT: FETAL HEART RATE:

BLOOD TEST RESULTS:

Checkup 4

DATE/TIME:

QUESTIONS TO ASK:

PRACTITIONER ADVICE/INSTRUCTIONS:

BLOOD PRESSURE: PULSE:

URINALYSIS: SUGAR: PROTEIN:

FUNDAL HEIGHT: FETAL HEART RATE:

BLOOD TEST RESULTS:

Checkup 5

DATE/TIME:

QUESTIONS TO ASK:

PRACTITIONER ADVICE/INSTRUCTIONS:

BLOOD PRESSURE: PULSE:

URINALYSIS: SUGAR: PROTEIN:

FUNDAL HEIGHT: FETAL HEART RATE:

BLOOD TEST RESULTS:

Checkup 6

DATE/TIME:

QUESTIONS TO ASK:

PRACTITIONER ADVICE/INSTRUCTIONS:

BLOOD PRESSURE: PULSE:

URINALYSIS: SUGAR: PROTEIN:

FUNDAL HEIGHT: FETAL HEART RATE:

BLOOD TEST RESULTS:

Checkup 7

DATE/TIME:

QUESTIONS TO ASK:

PRACTITIONER ADVICE/INSTRUCTIONS:

BLOOD PRESSURE: PULSE:

URINALYSIS: SUGAR: PROTEIN:

FUNDAL HEIGHT: FETAL HEART RATE:

BLOOD TEST RESULTS:

Checkup 8

DATE/TIME:

QUESTIONS TO ASK:

PRACTITIONER ADVICE/INSTRUCTIONS:

BLOOD PRESSURE: PULSE:

URINALYSIS: SUGAR: PROTEIN:

FUNDAL HEIGHT: FETAL HEART RATE:

BLOOD TEST RESULTS:

Checkup 9

DATE/TIME:

QUESTIONS TO ASK:

PRACTITIONER ADVICE/INSTRUCTIONS:

BLOOD PRESSURE: PULSE:

URINALYSIS: SUGAR: PROTEIN:

FUNDAL HEIGHT: FETAL HEART RATE:

BLOOD TEST RESULTS:

Checkup 10

DATE/TIME:

QUESTIONS TO ASK:

PRACTITIONER ADVICE/INSTRUCTIONS:

BLOOD PRESSURE: PULSE:

URINALYSIS: SUGAR: PROTEIN:

FUNDAL HEIGHT: FETAL HEART RATE:

BLOOD TEST RESULTS:

Checkup 11

DATE/TIME:

QUESTIONS TO ASK:

PRACTITIONER ADVICE/INSTRUCTIONS:

BLOOD PRESSURE: PULSE:

URINALYSIS: SUGAR: PROTEIN:

FUNDAL HEIGHT: FETAL HEART RATE:

BLOOD TEST RESULTS:

Checkup 12

DATE/TIME:

QUESTIONS TO ASK:

PRACTITIONER ADVICE/INSTRUCTIONS:

BLOOD PRESSURE: PULSE:

URINALYSIS: SUGAR: PROTEIN:

FUNDAL HEIGHT: FETAL HEART RATE:

BLOOD TEST RESULTS:

Checkup 13

DATE/TIME:

QUESTIONS TO ASK:

PRACTITIONER ADVICE/INSTRUCTIONS:

BLOOD PRESSURE: PULSE:

URINALYSIS: SUGAR: PROTEIN:

FUNDAL HEIGHT: FETAL HEART RATE:

BLOOD TEST RESULTS:

Checkup 14

DATE/TIME:

QUESTIONS TO ASK:

PRACTITIONER ADVICE/INSTRUCTIONS:

BLOOD PRESSURE: PULSE:

URINALYSIS: SUGAR: PROTEIN:

FUNDAL HEIGHT: FETAL HEART RATE:

BLOOD TEST RESULTS:

Checkup 15

DATE/TIME:

QUESTIONS TO ASK:

PRACTITIONER ADVICE/INSTRUCTIONS:

BLOOD PRESSURE: PULSE:

URINALYSIS: SUGAR: PROTEIN:

FUNDAL HEIGHT: FETAL HEART RATE:

BLOOD TEST RESULTS:

Checkup 16

DATE/TIME:

QUESTIONS TO ASK:

PRACTITIONER ADVICE/INSTRUCTIONS:

BLOOD PRESSURE: PULSE:

URINALYSIS: SUGAR: PROTEIN:

FUNDAL HEIGHT: FETAL HEART RATE:

BLOOD TEST RESULTS:

WEIGHT-GAIN RECORD

Intellectually, you know it: weight gain during pregnancy is a good thing, a sign that your baby is growing happily and healthfully inside you. But still, accepting that excess poundage can be tough, especially if, like most women, you've spent your entire life watching your weight.

One way to deal with this issue is simply to avoid looking at the scale. Sure, your practitioner must do frequent weight checks to monitor the baby's growth and to make sure you're gaining at an acceptable rate, but you're welcome to simply turn your head. Many women do this. Of course, others find pregnancy liberating when it comes to weight; for the first time in their lives, they can relax when they step on the scale. That's a great outlook. Just don't relax so much that you stop exercising and start eating a box of Oreos every morning.

However you feel about it, expect to gain 2 to 4 pounds during your first trimester, 3 to 5 pounds a month during the second trimester, and the bulk of your weight toward the end of your pregnancy. Everyone is different, though, so don't worry if you gain extra padding on the front end, as long as your doctor isn't concerned. Smaller women tend to gain more weight during the first few months of pregnancy.

Below are the American College of Obstetricians and Gynecologists guidelines for pregnancy weight gain. About half of women gain more weight than recommended, so ask your practitioner whether your prepregnancy weight was normal, underweight, or overweight and how much pregnancy weight gain is healthy for you. Because of the obesity epidemic, these guidelines may be revised in the near future.

PREPREGNANCY WEIGHT	RECOMMENDED WEIGHT GAIN
Underweight	28 to 40 pounds
Normal weight	25 to 35 pounds
Overweight	15 to 25 pounds

WEIGHT GAIN WEEK BY WEEK

Get an extra-large tape measure and wrap it around the largest diameter of your girth, typically right in line with your belly button.

WEEK	WEIGHT	BELLY SIZE
1		
2		
3		
4		
5		
6		
7		
8		
9		
10		
11		
12		
13		
14		
15		
16		
17		
18		
19		

WEEK	WEIGHT	BELLY SIZE
20		
21		
22		
23		
24		
25		
26		
27		
28		
29		
30		
31		
32		
33		
34		
35		
36		
37		
38		
39		
40		

TEST AND ULTRASOUND RESULTS

TEST DATE

RESULTS

_____

TEST DATE

RESULTS

_____

TEST DATE

RESULTS

_____

TEST DATE

RESULTS

_____

TEST DATE

RESULTS

_____

TEST DATE

RESULTS

_____

TEST AND ULTRASOUND RESULTS (continued)

TEST DATE

RESULTS

TEST DATE

RESULTS

TEST DATE

RESULTS

TEST DATE

RESULTS

TEST DATE

RESULTS

TEST DATE

RESULTS

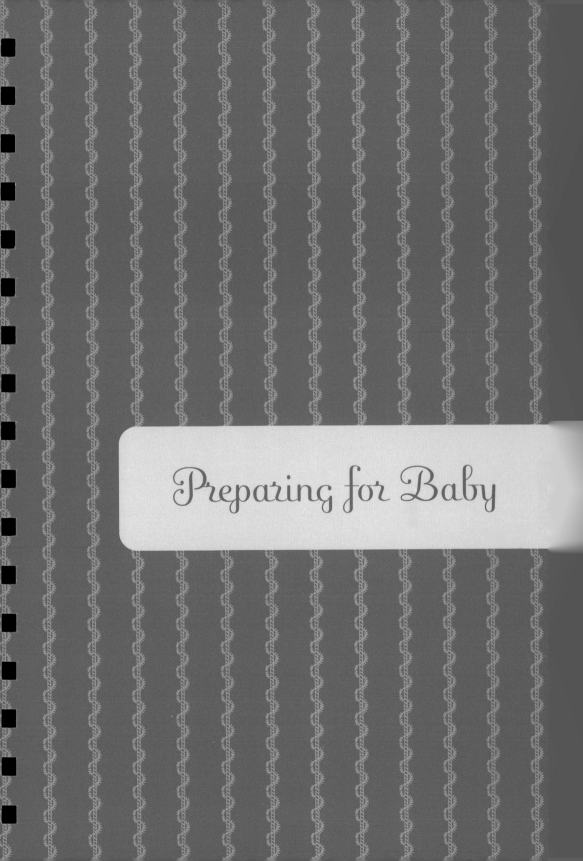

Preparing for Baby

Getting Ready for Baby

PLANNING AHEAD FOR BABY: A CHECKLIST

Once your baby is born, you will learn the meaning of the word *busy*. You think you understand it now, but once you add in the constant attention that your little one will demand and subtract several months' worth of sleep, you will come to appreciate the term in a whole new way. The trick is to buy some peace of mind by accomplishing as much as possible before the baby is born.

Use the checklist below to get ahead of the game. If you wait until after the baby arrives, you may find these tasks piling up, which will only add to your stress. Better to spend those first few weeks helping your baby adjust to the world than paying your electric bill.

This list is by no means comprehensive. We've pared it down to the easy-to-overlook essentials that, done in advance, will help you keep your sanity.

ONE TO TWO MONTHS BEFORE

☐ Pay bills in advance

☐ Sign will, insurance policies

☐ Set up bank accounts and college funds

☐ Sign up for cord-blood-bank service

☐ Confirm work/maternity-leave arrangements

☐ Get recommendations for babysitters, nannies, daycare providers

☐ Register for baby gifts

THREE WEEKS BEFORE

☐ Select birth announcements. (If you know the sex of your baby; if you don't, choose two so that you'll at least have it narrowed down before the baby arrives.)

☐ Address birth announcement and thank-you card envelopes

☐ Choose pediatrician

☐ Fill out insurance/medical forms

TWO WEEKS BEFORE

☐ Register at hospital

☐ Purchase baby first-aid supplies

☐ Purchase/rent breastfeeding equipment and supplies

ONE WEEK BEFORE

☐ Wash baby clothes

☐ Set up car seat

☐ Pack labor bag

☐ Pack hospital-stay and going-home bag

☐ Pack layette for baby

BABY NAMES IN CONTENTION

GIRL NAMES

BOY NAMES

BABY GIFTS AND THANK-YOU NOTES

GIFT	GIVER	NOTE SENT
		☐
		☐
		☐
		☐
		☐
		☐
		☐
		☐
		☐
		☐
		☐
		☐
		☐
		☐
		☐
		☐
		☐
		☐

GIFT	GIVER	NOTE SENT
		☐
		☐
		☐
		☐
		☐
		☐
		☐
		☐
		☐
		☐
		☐
		☐
		☐
		☐
		☐
		☐
		☐
		☐
		☐

Preparing for Delivery

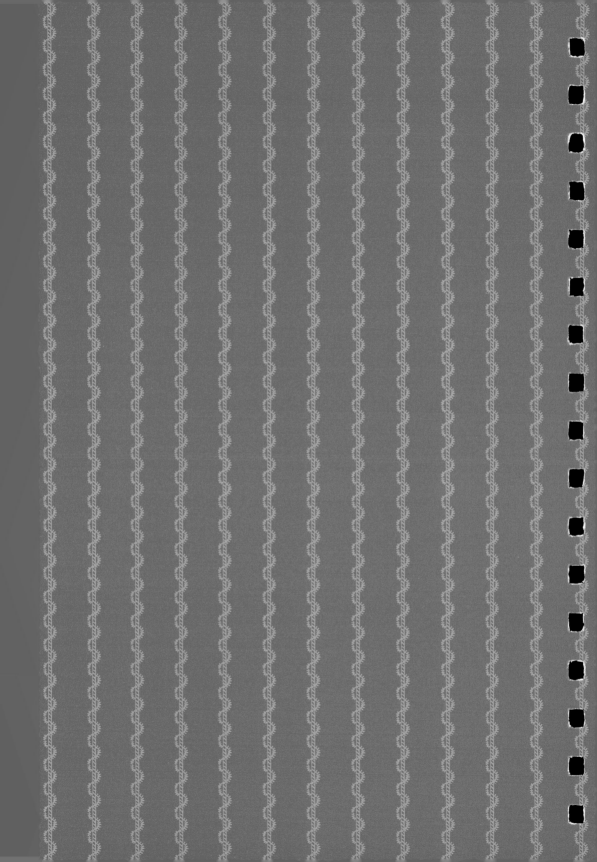

Preparing for Labor and Delivery

CHILDBIRTH CLASS NOTES

Attending a birthing class is probably the first time it's really, truly going to hit you: "I'm going to have a baby!"

This is a wonderful, happy feeling. It's also terrifying, because it's also going to hit you that this baby must come out of you one way or the other, and it's too late to do anything about it.

In birthing class, you get down to the nitty-gritty. You discuss ad nauseam what labor feels like and, worse, what it looks like. Chances are, you'll view several birth films, most of them a cross between those hokey high school health education films and *The Exorcist*. Some, like the one known in pregnancy circles as the "Brazilian Squatting film" (heaven knows what its real title is), are world-famous and quite graphic. As scary as all of this may seem to you, take heart in one of the immutable laws of pregnancy: it's your partner who will feel the queasiest and will be the most likely to pass out.

Don't worry. Take a deep breath—which, by the way, is one of the most valuable things you'll learn in class. You'll also learn how to make yourself more comfortable in the labor room, how to best use your birthing coach, and when, if you're considering that option, to ask for pain medication. It's also a good place to meet other couples who are in the same boat. Most women report feeling more emotionally and physically ready for the big event after taking classes.

CLASSMATE CONTACTS

NAME:

PHONE:

E-MAIL:

NAME:

PHONE:

E-MAIL:

NAME:

PHONE:

E-MAIL:

NAME:

PHONE:

E-MAIL:

NAME:

PHONE:

E-MAIL:

NAME:

PHONE:

E-MAIL:

WHAT TO BRING TO BIRTHING CLASS

- ☐ 2 large pillows

- ☐ birthing ball

- ☐ yoga mat

- ☐ camera

- ☐ snacks

- ☐ water

- ☐ pen for taking notes

BIRTHING CLASS NOTES

Class 1

DATE: _____   INSTRUCTOR: _____

TOPICS: _____

_____

NOTES: _____

_____

_____

_____

Class 2

DATE: _____   INSTRUCTOR: _____

TOPICS: _____

_____

NOTES: _____

_____

_____

_____

Class 3

DATE: _____   INSTRUCTOR: _____

TOPICS: _____

_____

NOTES: _____

_____

_____

_____

Class 4

DATE: _____ INSTRUCTOR: _____

TOPICS: _____

_____

NOTES: _____

_____

_____

_____

Class 5

DATE: _____ INSTRUCTOR: _____

TOPICS: _____

_____

NOTES: _____

_____

_____

_____

Class 6

DATE: _____ INSTRUCTOR: _____

TOPICS: _____

_____

NOTES: _____

_____

_____

_____

PACKING FOR THE BIG DAY

You probably won't actually need all this stuff, but there is some comfort in feeling prepared for anything. It's best to pack these items as three separate bags. In the birthing room, you're only going to want your labor paraphernalia; then let your partner take it away. In the hospital room, you'll want to keep baby's things separate from yours. In some hospitals, all the action may take place in a single room.

FOR BABY

☐ infant car seat

☐ newborn clothing: 2 onesies, 2 baby outfits, 2 pairs socks/booties, cap, jacket/snowsuit for winter babies

☐ 2 receiving blankets

☐ 1 swaddle blanket

☐ baby nail clippers

☐ diapers

☐ diaper bag

☐ bottles (if using)

FOR MOM IN LABOR

☐ workout/birthing ball

☐ relaxation/energizing items: music mixes (both energizing and relaxing), aromatherapy (both energizing and relaxing), massage oil, focal point such as a favorite picture

- [ ] pain relief: heat pack/pad, pillow, tennis ball, or rolling pin

- [ ] watch with second hand

- [ ] ponytail holder or scrunchie

- [ ] 2 pairs warm socks

- [ ] sweater or sweatshirt

- [ ] oversized T-shirt or nightdress

- [ ] blanket

- [ ] washcloth/towelettes

- [ ] toiletries: comb/brush, lip balm, small mirror

- [ ] lollipops/sucking candy

- [ ] snacks/drinks for your birthing coach

- [ ] cell phone or calling card and change for pay phone if cell phones aren't allowed

- [ ] change for vending machine

- [ ] camera/video camera

- [ ] pen

- [ ] magazines/books

- [ ] champagne or sparkling cider

FOR MOM'S HOSPITAL STAY

- ☐ medical insurance card
- ☐ ice packs
- ☐ spray-on pain relief
- ☐ seat doughnut
- ☐ hemorrhoid pads
- ☐ personal hygiene cleansing pads
- ☐ sanitary napkins
- ☐ pajamas
- ☐ bathrobe
- ☐ maternity/large pants
- ☐ maternity/large top
- ☐ nursing bra
- ☐ nursing pads
- ☐ extra underwear (large size)
- ☐ warm socks
- ☐ toiletries and makeup

CONTRACTIONS CHART

You may wonder if you'll know when you're having contractions. As any woman who's ever given birth will tell you: *you'll know.* When they start, they'll certainly grab your attention, not to mention your uterus.

There's no way to predict how forceful your contractions will be. Some women describe the experience as no worse than having bad gas, while others say their contractions feel like having someone operate a jackhammer inside their belly. Typically, contractions are milder when labor starts, and they grow longer, more intense, and more frequent as labor progresses.

How will you know when to call in the professionals? Discuss this in-depth with your medical practitioner, but once again: you'll know. As you're going through the experience, perhaps you can take comfort in the old adage, "It's the kind of pain you forget." It must be true. Otherwise no one would ever have more than one kid.

Use this chart to keep track of your labor pains. Bring it to your birthing place as a point of reference for your birthing team.

HEALTH PRACTITIONER'S PHONE: _____

BIRTH COACH PHONE: _____

BIRTH COACH PHONE: _____

TAXI OR CAR SERVICE PHONE: _____

START TIME OF CONTRACTION	END TIME OF CONTRACTION	CONTRACTION INTERVALS*	CONTRACTION INTENSITY

* Time between beginning of last contraction and start of most recent

START TIME OF CONTRACTION	END TIME OF CONTRACTION	CONTRACTION INTERVALS	CONTRACTION INTENSITY

START TIME OF CONTRACTION	END TIME OF CONTRACTION	CONTRACTION INTERVALS	CONTRACTION INTENSITY

Baby and Beyond

Meet Your Baby

NAME: _____

DATE OF BIRTH: _____

TIME OF BIRTH: _____

WEIGHT: _____

LENGTH: _____

HAIR COLOR: _____

ATTENDING DOCTOR OR MIDWIFE: _____

OTHERS PRESENT FOR DELIVERY: _____

_____

_____

_____

_____

Getting Your Body Back

Finally, you can see your feet again, even though the view looking down is a bit softer and squishier than it was before the baby. In most cases, if you had an uneventful pregnancy and labor, you can start back with some light activity such as walking or swimming within two weeks of giving birth. If you had a complicated pregnancy or a C-section, you may have to wait up to six or eight weeks before hitting the road again. Either way, before you race out the door, make sure your medical professional has given you the green light, and ramp up gradually. Even with the most uneventful pregnancy and delivery, a doctor's sign-off is important. Your body has just gone through a major event and needs a thorough checkup before you can test-drive it again.

Before you return to your official exercise program, you may want to do short bits of light activity right away—say, 5 or 10 minutes of walking the halls of the hospital—with your doctor's blessing, of course. At this point the goal shouldn't be weight loss or calorie burning but simply getting your body humming again.

Your body spent nine months stretching, growing, and changing, and it'll take about the same amount of time to get back to even close to where it was pre-baby. Breastfeeding, which burns about 500 calories a day, can help you lose weight, but the difference isn't huge—probably no more than 5 pounds over the course of a year—because when you're nursing you also eat more. When it comes to postpartum weight loss, your eating habits and physical activity level play a more important role in weight loss than whether or not you nurse your baby. Keep in mind, too, that your body needs to be slightly heavier for milk production; many active women report returning to near, or even below, their pre-baby weight as soon as they stop breastfeeding.

It may take several months for your stamina and strength to approach your prepregnancy levels, but if you exercised throughout your pregnancy, you'll bounce back a lot more quickly than if you didn't. And if you're an athlete or serious exerciser, take heart: you have the capacity to retain—or even exceed—

your previous fitness level. Plenty of elite runners have gone on to win races and set personal records after giving birth. In the 1996 Olympics, Svetlana Masterkova of Russia won the 800-meter and 1,500-meter races about a year after delivering a daughter, then broke the world record for the mile a few months later.

In fact, some research suggests that the combination of exercise and pregnancy may have a greater training effect than exercise alone, probably due to the increase in blood volume and changing hormone levels. In other words, the adaptations your body must make to carry the extra—and constantly increasing—load may, in some respects, simulate a workout. Studies of avid exercisers suggest that their aerobic capacity improves by 5 to 10 percent after pregnancy, an effect that becomes most apparent six months to one year after delivery.

Still, it's going to take awhile to feel—and perform—like yourself again. You may be in for some surprises when you first lace up. On the upside, you'll be so much lighter when you're moving that you'll almost feel like a feather being blown in the breeze. You'll also have fewer parts of your body flapping, flouncing, and bouncing with every step.

On the other hand, your bladder may leak when you exert yourself to the point of heavy breathing. Your abdominal muscles may feel strained, and your breathing may feel a bit out of whack. All of this is normal, even the lack of bladder control. Some of these setbacks will last just a few workouts, while others may take a few months to subside.

If possible, find an exercise class geared toward new moms so that you can work out alongside women going through the same struggles you are. Or, if postnatal classes aren't available near you, look for a mom's group where women swap babysitting duties and exercise DVDs so that everyone gets to work out.

You may feel more comfortable hiring a personal trainer for a few sessions to jump-start your journey back to fitness. Be sure to choose a trainer who is experienced in postnatal exercise. You might even consider seeking out a nurse, physical therapist, or midwife who is also certified as a personal trainer by the American Council on Exercise, American College of Sports Medicine, or National Strength and Conditioning Association. Setting an exercise goal, such as running a 5k or completing a certain hike, can help motivate you. Just be sure to set realistic expectations. Planning a 100-mile bike ride three months after you've given birth probably isn't the most sensible goal.

Two of the biggest hurdles you'll have when trying to get back into shape are lack of time and lack of sleep. It's awfully tough to get motivated for intervals on the treadmill when you've gotten up for the midnight, 3 A.M., and 6 A.M. feedings. This is the time to resort to a trick you might have used when you were pregnant: adding up short bouts of exercise throughout the day. Don't be shy about asking for help. Hopefully your partner will be so in awe of your strength during pregnancy and labor — and so beholden to you for bringing this wonderful child into your lives — that he or she won't mind carving out an hour of sweat time for you a few days a week.

GEAR TO GET BACK IN SHAPE

Here are some helpful items to help you get back in shape. This list is in addition to the prenatal workout gear on page 27. You might need to buy some of those items again, depending on how beat up they are from supporting nine months of extra weight.

- ☐ baby jogger stroller

- ☐ baby carrier/Bjorn

- ☐ active-mom diaper bag (a hands-free design that slings over the shoulder so you can use it when you walk or hike)

- ☐ yoga mat

- ☐ bands and/or weights

- ☐ tune belt/fanny pack/armband

WHERE TO BUY POSTPARTUM WORKOUT GEAR

| www.lizlange.com | www.tinyride.com | www.terrysports.com |
| www.title9sports.com | www.lucy.com | www.activasports.com |
